Doctors & Doctrines

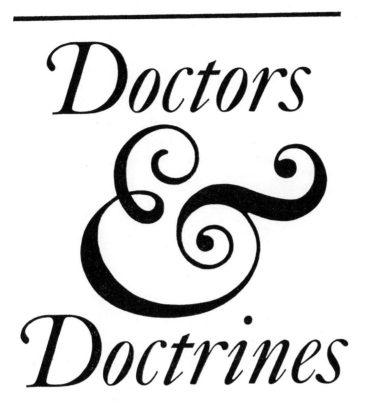

Doctors & Doctrines

THE IDEOLOGY OF MEDICAL CARE IN CANADA

Bernard R. Blishen

UNIVERSITY OF TORONTO PRESS

© University of Toronto Press 1969

Printed in Canada

SBN 8020 1614 6 (cloth) / 8020 6105 2 (paper)

For Ruth

PREFACE

MUCH HAS BEEN written concerning the medical profession's reaction to medical care insurance administered and financed by government. The Canadian Medical Association, in periodic official statements, has sought to specify the profession's stand on medical care insurance by indicating the characteristics of the type of plan which in its view protects the interests of the public and the profession. Those who believe in greater government involvement in the organization, administration, and financing of medical care insurance have claimed that the profession's reaction has been based mainly on professional self-interests. The public and professional debate on this issue was intensified by the 1962 medicare dispute in Saskatchewan and the publication in 1964 of volumes I and II of the *Report* of the Royal Commission on Health Services.

This book is an attempt to examine the statements of the medical profession in Canada concerning the public and professional implications of medical care insurance as part of an ideological reaction to the strains which physicians face in a changing social and medical world. The ideology of medicine no doubt embraces many more propositions than those specified in the profession's statements on medical care insurance. However, since administrative and financial control by government of this type of insurance could have such far-reaching consequences for the freedom and autonomy of the medical profession, it is highly probable that the most fundamental ideological propositions are contained in these statements. Physicians maintain this ideology because the propositions, themes, and values it contains helps them to overcome the doubts and anxieties engendered by the strain and conflict they encounter in their professional roles.

My interest in the functional implications of what physicians and their representatives say about medical care insurance was aroused during my association with the Royal Commission on Health Services as its Research Director. Volumes I and II of the Commission's *Report* attempted to answer the claims and allay the fears of the medical profession concerning the introduction of medical care insurance in a reasoned and rational manner. The reaction of the spokesmen for the profession to the Commission's argument suggests that this attempt failed in its purpose. This study seeks to provide some reasons for the continued concern of the medical profession, which in some provinces must now actually practice under the conditions of a government-sponsored medical care insurance scheme, and in others faces a similar prospect in the future.

Much of the factual material used in this study was collected by the Royal Commission on Health Services for the purpose of studying a range of problems associated with the organization of health care. That these data can be used at all in this study is thus fortuitous rather than planned.

I am grateful to a number of organizations and individuals for their encouragement and assistance. The award of a fellowship from the Laidlaw Foundation in 1964 allowed me to begin this study. I should point out, however, that publication of a study supported by a Laidlaw Foundation fellowship does not imply responsibility of the Foundation for the content of the study, or agreement with the opinions expressed; these are properly the responsibility of the author. Trent University provided assistance in a number of ways, and I am particularly grateful to President T. H. B. Symons for his consideration in allowing me the time required to undertake this study at a time when all his efforts, and those of my academic colleagues, were directed to the launching of the first academic year of this new University. Professor J. C. McDonald of Trent University and Dr. Wendell Macleod of the Canadian Association of Medical Schools read the manuscript and made valuable comments. The final manuscript was greatly improved by the careful editing of Miss Francess Halpenny of the University of Toronto Press. Dr. Alice Martin and my students, Robert Korth, Susan McBride, Rick Nichols, and Tony Arthur, worked at various times as research assistants. Joanne Heath patiently typed and retyped the manscript, at times assisted by Marilyn Metcalfe.

B. B.

CONTENTS

TABLES

Doctors & Doctrines

I

INTRODUCTION

THE DIFFICULTIES facing organized medicine today must be seen against the background of the social change occurring in our society. This change affects the various arrangements through which medicine is practised, with resulting pressure and strain upon the physician. It is true, of course, that although much of present-day social change gives the appearance of disorganization and chaos there is, nevertheless, an underlying order to many of our daily activities. Seemingly, while many significant elements in our social structure change rapidly, others do so at a much slower rate and thereby tend to support the individual as he seeks to adjust to the apparent chaos. But the process of adjustment produces tensions and strains both within the individual and within the institutions of which he is part. He can react to these tensions in a number of ways. It should be stressed that this study is limited to the analysis of only one type of reaction, the ideological. It seeks to show the difficulties facing the physician today as he attempts to meet the demands of his professional role, and his reaction to these difficulties in terms of his professional ideology. That ideology functions as a socially acceptable means of overcoming the emotional conflicts, anxieties, and doubts which he faces as he seeks to practise his skills in a rapidly changing world.

The focus of this analysis is the physician's role, but this is only one, albeit a crucial one, in a wide range of roles which comprise the total medical care system. Certain combinations of these roles are organized into sub-systems which include medical schools, hospitals, practice in its various organizational forms such as solo, partnership, and group practice, professional associations, and third party arrangements for financing medical care.

Since the medical care system is an integral part of society, the relationship between them is reciprocal; changes in medical care may have repercussions for the structure of society. Changes of this type will not be studied as part of this analysis, but one example is the growth of arrangements for prepaying the costs of medical care by governments and other third parties, which make early access to medical care possible for greater numbers of people whose illnesses are thereby shortened in length and whose productivity is retained for a longer period. The economic productivity of society is thus increased. Another example is found in the changes in treatment of certain types of diseases. As medicine conquers the diseases of the young, the larger number of survivors of the early years of life enter the educational system thus creating pressures for change in techniques of instruction at all levels of education in order to handle the increased inflow of students.[1] Subsequently, this larger body of students enters the labour force and their entry also increases the economic productivity of society.

But change, as we have said, is not a one way street. Social change can generate pressure for change in the system of medical care. The growth of scientific knowledge, demographic change, higher educational levels, changing social values, and changes in family structure all have an impact on the structure of the various parts of the medical care system which can create serious strains in the physician's role. Subsequent chapters will focus on various aspects of the relationship between these strains and the parts of the medical care system. Before turning to this task, however, a brief general discussion is required to show the manner in which wider social changes can effect changes in the medical care system.

One of the main features of social change today is the increasingly rapid rate in the growth of scientific knowledge. Paradoxically, while our social values stimulate scientific activity, especially scientific innovation, and many of our social arrangements depend on the successful functioning of science, its success, particularly in its technical and utilitarian application, tends to weaken certain social values and the social arrangements based upon them.

In all societies man has sought to master his environment by effectively fitting means to ends, whether these ends be empirical or non-empirical. Western society has emphasized empirical ends, although this concern has not excluded the non-empirical. The choice of means for particular ends follows the dictates of rational thought; that is, according to the canons of Aristotelian logic.[2] Rationality in Western society is widely

1 / Some indication of the effect of the application of new medical knowledge in the treatment of disease is provided by Kohn. His estimate, based on the application of the 1926 death rate for the period 1926–61, indicates that the Canadian population increased by 1,067,000 during that period owing to the decline in mortality. R. Kohn, *The Health of the Canadian People*, Royal Commission on Health Services, Ottawa: Queen's Printer, 1967, p. 128.

2 / Bernard Barber, *Science and the Social Order*, Glencoe, Ill.: The Free Press, 1952, p. 8.

approved and institutionalized not only in scientific activities but also in other activities as well. "... rationality, wherever manifested, has the same effect of producing changes and of undermining established routines. Social instability is in part, then, the price we pay for our institutionalization of rationality."[3]

The growth of medical knowledge creates difficulties for the medical educator and the practising physician in developing the medical school's curriculum. The former must insert new knowledge into the curriculum, by adding material and sometimes by replacing older knowledge which is supported by entrenched academic interests. But the rapid expansion of the subject-matter to be mastered by the modern medical student means that in comparison with previous generations of students he is expected to learn more, although with less possibility of doing so. The realization of his increasingly limited capacity to grasp the expanding body of medical knowledge promotes feelings of uncertainty within the student which he carries with him into practice. These feelings may be accentuated as knowledge grows, but the pressures of practice tend to frustrate any hopes he may have of trying to keep up-to-date with it.

Perhaps the most obvious of all social changes evident in the contemporary world, and Canada is no exception, is the rapid increase in population, which has a direct effect on the demand for medical care and on its availability. Although the rate of population growth varies between countries and regions of the world, there is, nevertheless, an absolute increase in numbers. At the beginning of this century Canada's population was just over 5 million; sixty-one years later it was nearly three times as large and according to the estimates prepared by the Royal Commission on Health Services, by 1991 it will probably be between 35 and 37 million.[4] An indication of the effect of population growth on the demand for medical services is provided by the Commission which showed that

Over the thirty-five year period 1926–1961, when expenditures on personal health services grew at a trend rate of 6.7 percent, population growth accounted for 1.9 percentage points – approximately 30 percent of total growth ... but its effect was most significant in the period before 1945. ... Thus, in the years 1926–1944, when the trend rate of growth of total spending was 2 percent per year, 1.3 percentage points (almost two thirds of total growth) was attributable to population change. In the years 1945–1961, although population increase now accounted for 2.6 percentage points, it only accounted for about one quarter of the total growth rate of 11.8 percent.[5]

3 / *Ibid.*, p. 211.
4 / Royal Commission on Health Services, *Final Report*, vol. I, Ottawa: Queen's Printer, 1964, p. 112.
5 / *Ibid.*, pp. 450–54.

Of particular significance in any analysis of the social changes which have occurred in Canada is the extent to which the population tends to migrate from rural to urban areas. In the sixty years between 1901 and 1961 Canada has changed from a predominantly rural to a predominantly urban population. In 1901 the percentage of our population living in rural areas stood at 62.5, but by 1961 this had declined to 39.3. On the other hand, the percentage of the population living in urban areas moved from 37.5 to 60.7 during this period.[6]

Kasahara has shown that between 1951 and 1961 the population of Canada's seventeen metropolitan areas increased by more than 2.5 milion or 45 per cent, or more than twice the growth rate of non-metropolitan areas.[7] With few exceptions this was a growth of suburban population, half of which was due to the excess of in-migration over out-migration.

Urbanization tends to draw a disproportionate share of physicians into urban centres to meet the demand of urban dwellers for medical services. This is particularly obvious in Canada's large metropolitan areas. For example, in 1961, Halifax, with 25 per cent of the provincial population, had 47.9 per cent of the physicians practising in Nova Scotia; Montreal, with 40.1 per cent of the provincial population, had 60.5 per cent of the physicians practising in the Province of Quebec; Toronto, with 29.3 per cent of the provincial population, had 39.3 per cent of the physicians practising in Ontario; Winnipeg, with 51.6 per cent of the provincial population, had 79.2 per cent of the physicians practising in Manitoba; and Vancouver, with 48.5 per cent of the provincial population, had 62.9 per cent of the physicians practising in British Columbia.[8]

The growth of scientific knowledge and innovation and population growth and movement are accompanied by a change in the social values and beliefs which underlie human behaviour. Some values remain unspoken assumptions, but they nevertheless guide behaviour. Other values, on the other hand, are institutionalized in that they provide explicit rules and procedures which have moral significance. The gradual erosion of elitism and the strengthening of equalitarianism are an example of change in social values. Lipset claims that "in the United States the effective emphasis on achievement and on equality of opportunity is reflected by the demands of lower status individuals for access to education as a means to success, and the recognition by the privileged that education as a means

6 / Dominion Bureau of Statistics, *Census of Canada, 1961*, vol. I, part 1, Ottawa: Queen's Printer, 1963, Table 12.

7 / Yoshiko Kasahara, "A Profile of Canada's Metropolitan Centres," in B. R. Blishen *et al.* (eds.), *Canadian Society*, 2nd ed., Toronto: Macmillan Co., 1964, pp. 53–62.

8 / S. Judek, *Medical Manpower in Canada*, Royal Commission on Health Services, Ottawa: Queen's Printer, 1964, p. 134.

to success must be given to all who are qualified. By contrast, in Canada education has had a more elitist and ascriptive import."[9] Porter emphasizes the elitist nature of Canadian society and claims that little has been done to change the structure of educational institutions in which these values are embedded, and which restrict equality of educational opportunity.[10] Although Lipset and Porter may be correct in their claims, there is ample evidence available which indicates that in Canada elitism as a significant value in the structure of our educational institutions is weakening. The decline is due, in part, to the fact that modern industry cannot operate effectively without the rational use of labour. Rational use requiries that ability and skill be recognized rather than family status, religion, and other ascriptive characteristics. The exploitation of the individual's ability becomes one of the major purposes of society's educational institutions, and to serve the demands of modern industrial society these institutions must be open to all with the ability to profit by them without social, economic, or cultural restrictions. The principle of equality of opportunity and the principle of the rational use of economic resources tend to be mutually reinforcing providing the educational system recognizes ability.[11] Individual abilities can then be matched with the occupational and professional needs of the economy through the market mechanisms of demand and supply.

The extent to which equality of educational opportunity still remains to be achieved in Canada is evident from census data. In 1961, in those families in which the family head earned under $3,000 per year, about 61 per cent of the children between 15 and 18 years of age, and 12 per cent of those between 19 and 24 years of age, were at school. But in those families in which the family head earned $7,000 and over per year, nearly 91 per cent of the 15 to 18 age group and 50 per cent of the 19 to 24 age group were at school. This same source also reveals that those in high-salaried managerial and professional occupations have a much higher proportion of their children in school in both these age groups than those in the low-salaried wage-earning occupations.[12]

These existing differences tend to obscure the fact that significant changes have occurred in the extent of educational opportunity in Canada, and that these changes have resulted in a higher level of education gener-

9 / S. M. Lipset, *Revolution and Counter-Revolution: The United States and Canada,* Berkeley: Institute of International Studies, University of California, reprint no. 193, 1965, p. 24.

10 / John Porter, *The Vertical Mosaic,* Toronto: University of Toronto Press, 1965, p. 167.

11 / *Ibid.*

12 / Dominion Bureau of Statistics, *Census of Canada, 1961,* Ottawa: Queen's Printer, 1963, Bulletin 7.1–10, Table 10.

ally in the population. In 1961, of the population 15 years of age and over not attending school, the percentage with no schooling rose from 1.1 in the 15 to 19 age group to 4.8 in the age group 65 and over. In other words, the proportion of the population with no schooling is steadily declining.[13] An increase in the proportions of the population completing the various levels of education in succeeding generations is also evident. In 1961 just over 30 per cent of the 20–24 age group completed no more than elementary education, but this proportion represents less than half the nearly 64 per cent of the age group 65 and over with no more than this level of education. On the other hand, a secondary level of education was the highest level of schooling of a far higher proportion of the younger age groups than of the older age groups: nearly 64 per cent of the 20 to 24 years olds compared with just under 28 per cent of the age group 65 and over.

Another significant change in values which is becoming increasingly evident today is the weakening of individualism embodied in the "free-enterprise" ideology, and the strengthening of collectivism which is evident in the increasing role of government in our daily lives. Although *laissez-faire* values have always been a significant feature of Canadian business enterprise, they have not assumed the importance given to them in the United States. That they have not is owing, in part at least, to the necessity for government intervention in national development in Canada. In the past, the national aspirations of this country were threatened by revolutionary ideas, military adventures, and economic competition from south of its border. If Canada was to become a nation these threats had to be met with specific government action although *laissez-faire* principles remained paramount. Through a variety of means such as public expenditures, transfer payments, subsidies, taxes and tariffs, and monetary policies, successive governments of Canada have played a significant role in national development both social and economic. That role has been particularly obvious since the depression and World War II, both of which required government intervention especially in economic affairs. Today *laissez-faire* principles are under severe pressure. The public appears to be increasingly disposed towards government intervention and control of the business world which is the seat of these values. It no longer considers the independent operation of market forces as the major secular arbiter of man's fate.[14] The role of government is to meet the many new – and

13 / *Ibid.*, Table 17.
14 / Survey results reveal that in the eleven-year period prior to 1965 public support for private ownership of industry has dropped from 68.6 per cent to 60.7 per cent. *Globe and Mail*, Toronto, November 19, 1965.

old – social and economic needs. These needs arise as social changes create society-wide problems, and it requires the power and resources of government to meet them. As the Royal Commission on Health Services points out:

Democratic government is an agency which enables us to transcend exclusively individual and selfish drives and to provide benefits for all, or at least a majority, of the nation's individuals. Many different arrangements have been developed to implement economic and social policies, the result of a complex process of discussion, negotiation, voting, decision making and budgeting. Throughout this procedure there is an emphasis upon finding out what is the overriding national interest and to discover the means for achieving acceptable solutions in the interdependent society of today.[15]

Underlying much of the increased government activity, especially in the field of health, welfare, and education, is a strengthened humanitarian concern. Humanitarianism is an essential component of our value system, but the extent to which governments base policies on this principle waxes and wanes. Two world wars and a great depression have resulted in its present emphasis especially in the three fields already mentioned. However, the emphasis on humanitarianism is accompanied by an attempt to rationalize it in economic terms. This takes the form of analyses of what is termed "investment in human capital." Expenditures for health, for example, are claimed to result in a larger productive labour force "by extending the length of working life and by ensuring that individuals are able to work more regularly during their productive years."[16] Again quoting the Royal Commission on Health Services,

Expenditures on health services are, in many cases, quite different from the purchase of an ordinary consumer good. They may actually be a form of investment in human capital; they may be more important in an affluent society, than additional expenditures on food and shelter and they may yield important external benefits for the family and the society as a whole. If income is not a barrier to purchase health services we can expect that a significant proportion of individual or family resources will be devoted to their purchase.[17]

These changing social values have affected the medical care system. For example, the increased emphasis on equality of opportunity in Canada, particularly equality of educational opportunity, has resulted in higher education levels which is manifested in the growth of literacy. Information about the advances in medical knowledge is widely disseminated by the mass media throughout the population which, being more

15 / Royal Commission on Health Services, *Final Report*, vol. i, pp. 771–72.
16 / *Ibid.*, p. 501.
17 / *Ibid.*, p. 508.

literate than previous generations, is more aware of medicine's power to heal and more critical of the quality of medical care. Thus, higher educational levels have generated an increased volume of care, the aggregate effect of the propensity of individuals to consume increasing amounts of health care. Further, the increased importance given to collectivism in Canadian society has encouraged the emergence of a public, as opposed to a private, approach to the solution of the problem of the availability of and payment for medical services, as well as an increasing emphasis on these services as a "civic right." These latter value changes have resulted in the introduction of public measures to pay the cost of medical services. Without an economic barrier to the consumption of these services, the individual tends to increase his consumption of them up to a certain level. This increase creates pressure upon the physician to meet the demands of a growing number of patients who want medical care of the highest quality.

The changing pattern of individual consumption of health services is described by the Royal Commission on Health Services thus:

Per capita expenditures on health services have increased rapidly over the whole period 1926–1961 both because average consumption has increased and because the prices of individual health services have risen.... over these thirty-five years the value of personal health services received by each Canadian rose fivefold from $17.59 to $88.41, while if prescribed drugs are included the sum amounted to $94.52 in the latter year.[18]

Part of this increase is due to increases in the prices of the various health services. Despite these price increases, however, "the average Canadian more than doubled his consumption of personal health services during this period."[19] Although prices affect the consumption of health services, between 1945 and 1961 their effect tended to diminish while per capita consumption increased. "In the years 1950–1954, of a total increase of 10.9 per cent a year, the rise due to price change was 5.7 percentage points. In the period 1957–61, out of a total growth rate of 10.3 the rise due to price change was 2.5 percentage points."[20] Recent data indicate that in the period 1957–67 the average annual rate of growth of the Consumer Price Index was 2.0 per cent compared with 3.1 per cent for the health care component.[21]

In an attempt to provide an increased supply of physicians and thereby relieve the pressure which increased per capita consumption of medical

18 / *Ibid.*, p. 454.
19 / *Ibid.*
20 / *Ibid.*, p. 455.
21 / Canada, Department of National Health and Welfare, *Health Care Price Movements*, Ottawa: 1968, mimeo.

services places on the physician, society has created new medical schools, expanded existing ones, and facilitated the inflow of foreign-born physicians. According to Judek,

The number of physicians between 1911 and 1931 did not keep pace with the growth of the Canadian population and hence in 1931 there were more people per physician (1:1,034) than in 1911 (1:972). This trend has been reversed since 1931 and the national physician–population ratio has steadily improved to 1:968 in 1948 and 1:857 in 1961.[22]

This improvement has continued and by 1965 the ratio stood at 1:833.[23] To a large extent the improvement is due to large numbers of immigrant physicians coming to Canada to practise.

The considerable improvement in the national physician–population ratio between 1951 and 1961 was due to a great inflow of immigrant doctors during those years. Out of nearly 15,000 newly registered physicians in Canada during the years 1950–60, about one third were immigrant physicians. Over the same years, the immigrant doctors were equal to about one-half of the total output of 9,300 graduates of Canadian medical schools.[24]

Some evidence exists that despite the improvement in the physician–population ratio the increase in per capita consumption of medical services has increased the work load of the individual physician. Using data obtained from a questionnaire survey of physicians in Canada, Judek reports that in 1962 the weekly working hours per doctor ranged from around 50 to just over 52, depending on the type of practice: solo, partnership, or group.[25] Six years later preliminary results of a survey of physicians undertaken by the Canadian Medical Association indicate that the average hours worked per week in 1967 ranged from 61 to nearly 63 depending on the size of the community in which the physician practised.[26] The increased work load of the physician is reflected in the rise in his income. Income data based on taxation statistics published by the Department of National Health and Welfare reveal that in the years 1962 to 1965 the average net earnings of active fee-practice physicians rose from $16,970 to $22,064, an increase of 30 per cent.[27]

Changes in the structure of the family have affected the manner in which health services are provided. Rural-urban movement and the

22 / Judek, *Medical Manpower in Canada*, p. 8.
23 / Data supplied by the Department of National Health and Welfare.
24 / Judek, p. 9.
25 / *Ibid.*, p. 344.
26 / Canadian Medical Association, *Preliminary Results of C.M.A. and Provincial Licensing Authority: Survey of Canadian Medical Manpower*, 1967, mimeo.
27 / Data supplied by Department of National Health and Welfare.

geographic mobility of the population generally loosen traditional family ties. The family head, seeking to sell his occupational skills where the demand is high and the rewards are greatest, must retain a degree of geographic mobility if he is to get the best return for his labour. Such mobility usually means movement from one urban concentration to another. In each one the individual establishes social contacts beyond the confines of the traditional family with its network of kin. But the weight of numbers in these urban concentrations results in a greater complexity in human relationships which are, at the same time, more fleeting and impersonal for the most part. The weakening of the ties of the wider kinship group has resulted in the emergence of the small, relatively isolated modern family usually dependent for the satisfaction of its consumption needs on the income of the father. Because of its relative isolation from related kin who in earlier periods could support it in time of stress, and because of the present-day technical complexity of the services required to meet many of its needs, the family has relinquished many of its functions to more specialized social institutions. One of these is the hospital.

In our society values are changing and the educational level of the population is rising. These changes generate on the one hand a demand for medical care as a "civic right" and on the other an increasingly critical attitude towards the care provided. The physician, who is seeking to provide an increasing amount of care in spite of the difficulties he faces in mastering the growing corpus of medical knowledge and the anxieties which this situation generates, more and more uses the facilities of the modern hospital for the care of his patients. There can be little doubt that, if accurate data were available, it would be evident that at the turn of the century the incidence of hospitalization was much lower, and the proportion of the sick cared for by the family was much higher, than they are today. Recent data show the continuation of this trend towards higher incidence of hospitalization. During the period 1948–66 admissions to public general hospitals rose from 111 to 152 per thousand population. These rates are even higher than those for similar types of hospitals in the more affluent United States where admissions during the same period rose from 105 to 140 per thousand population. In fact, in this period Canada has had a higher number of beds per thousand population, and a higher number of days of hospital care per thousand population as well as a higher average length of hospital stay per admission than the United States.[28]

28 / Louis S. Reed and Willine Carr, "Utilization and Cost of General Hospital Care: Canada and the United States, 1948–66," *United States Social Security Bulletin*, November 1968, pp. 12–20.

This brief introduction has illustrated the manner in which social change has affected the system of medical care. It is the changes in the elements of that system – the medical school, the hospital, the organization of practice, the professional association, and third party arrangements – which are associated with role strains. Before discussing the nature of that association, however, we must attempt to set forth the theoretical framework to be used for this purpose and specify the meaning of the concepts *profession, role, role strain,* and *ideology.*

2

SOME THEORETICAL
ASSUMPTIONS

FOR THEIR CONTINUED economic growth, modern societies depend upon the technical application of an increasing body of scientific knowledge. One of the hallmarks of modernity is the rate of increase in this corpus of knowledge but since the boundaries of the corpus are beyond any one individual's ability to encompass, application of knowledge today requires specialization and a division of labour of which the professions are an integral part. As members of a profession, individuals perform specialized roles in relation to clientele. In so doing they encounter certain strains; these in part, are resolved both verbally and symbolically by the reiteration of the basic values, or themes, which shape the professional ideology.

PROFESSIONS AND PROFESSIONAL ROLES

Although the application of new industrial techniques requires individuals with special training in these fields, particular techniques may exist without the emergence of a profession. But as the numbers of individuals practising a particular technical role increase, a consciousness of purpose emerges amongst them which may eventually lead to a formal professional organization. Originally such organizations, based on the realization of the similarity of the technical roles its members performed, were study groups, or societies, whose purpose was to promote discussion, research, and publication in a particular technical field. As specialized roles emerged they were given titles which only those performing them were allowed to wear. For those who performed these roles the titles carried symbolic meaning in terms of the individual's identity and self-image.

Kinds of work tend to be named, to become well defined occupations, and an important part of a person's work based identity grows out of his relationship to his occupational title. These names carry a great deal of symbolic meaning, which tends to be incorporated into the identity. In the first place, they specify an area of endeavour belonging to those bearing the name and locate this area in relation to similar kinds of activity in a broader field. Secondly, they imply a great deal about the characteristics of their bearers, and these meanings are often systematized into elaborate ideologies which itemize the qualities, interests and capabilities of those so identified.[1]

In order to protect their technical titles and to distinguish the degree of competence which they implied, the early professional societies restricted membership to those who could prove their competence. This was done through examinations which became part of a licensing system. Besides the recognition of technical competence, professional societies sought to protect the public from dishonourable practitioners through the formulation of ethical codes.[2] In addition, "it became obvious that a relatively high level of remuneration implies a public recognition of status, and that the most certain way of attaining the latter is to press for the former. Hence protective activities are added to those already mentioned."[3]

Present-day professions have emerged from these developments. Before being admitted to a profession recruits are required by its professional licensing body to undertake a course of studies in professionally recognized training institutions, which may be part of a university. The practical application of the body of knowledge gained through the course of studies requires the acquisition of skills. Professional training, therefore, is both an intellectual and a practical preparation. It is his acquisition of the body of knowledge and professional skills, both of which his client lacks, that gives the professional his authority. This authority is given public recognition both formal and informal.

A non-professional occupation has customers who are presumed to know what goods or services they want. This knowledge includes their ability to judge the extent to which the goods or services will satisfy their wants. In this sense, "the customer is always right." In a profession, however, the determination of the client's needs is the responsibility of the professional, a responsibility based upon his superior knowledge. Because he lacks this knowledge, the client cannot judge the quality of the professional services he receives or the competence of the person providing them. In fact, the client surrenders to professional authority thus giving the professional a monopoly in his specific field of service, but in no other.

A profession possesses the means of maintaining technical and ethical standards; it is given the authority to do so through legislation to discipline members, at least to a degree. These legal privileges serve to protect the public, but they also add to the public prestige of the profession.

1 / H. S. Becker and J. Carper, "The Elements of Identification with an Occupation," *American Sociological Review*, vol. 21, no. 3, June 1956, pp. 341–47.

2 / A. M. Carr-Saunders and P. A. Wilson, *The Professions*, new ed., London: Frank Cass, 1964, pp. 298–304.

3 / *Ibid.*, p. 303.

The influence of any profession on public policy depends on its prestige. If the public image of the profession is harmed, its influence will decline. However, the extent of this influence also depends on the degree to which the professional group is organized for action in pursuit of its own, or the public's, interests; on the competence of its leaders; and on the value which the public places on the services which the profession has to offer.[4]

The norms of a professional group are contained in its code of ethics which governs behaviour in social situations. The code is an attempt to provide a statement of the service responsibilities of its members and at the same time it makes it possible for them to pursue their legitimate economic interests.[5] The code also incorporates the generally accepted values of the community and applies them to the particular sphere of interest of the profession so that members are aware of their responsibilities to the community. In this way, the community maintains a degree of control over the professions. The code also defines the appropriate behaviour of members of the profession towards each other, towards their clients, and towards unauthorized practitioners.[6]

The definitions in any code are based on certain broad general principles. A professional has an obligation to serve according to the best of his ability. He must maintain professional secrecy since he is privy to the confidence of his client. He must be financially disinterested in the advice he gives others. He cannot enter into economic competition with his professional colleagues. Competition is only allowed in terms of reputation for ability, which means that he cannot offer cheap lines for slender purses, advertise, or use other methods of competition evident in the business world. Lastly, he cannot allow unqualified persons to practise for him.[7]

The control over professional conduct exerted by the code of ethics is necessary because of the nature of the relationship between professional and client. In this relationship, the professional, because of his superior knowledge and skill, has an advantage over the client which is open to exploitation. This advantage is particularly evident in the doctor-patient relationship. The prestige accorded to the professions by the public is a recognition of the fact that although the opportunity for exploitation exists the professional typically refuses it.[8] In the contemporary world these opportunities are increasing, and if the professions are to retain the

4 / H. F. Gosnell and M. J. Schmidt, "Professional Associations," *Annals of the American Academy of Political and Social Science*, vol. 179, May 1935, p. 26.

5 / R. M. MacIver, "The Social Significance of Professional Ethics," *Annals of the American Academy of Political and Social Science*, vol. 297, January 1955, pp. 120–24.

6 / William J. Goode, "Community within a Community: The Professions," *American Sociological Review*, vol. 22, no. 2, April 1957, pp. 194–200.

7 / Carr-Saunders and Wilson, *The Professions*, pp. 421–24.

8 / Goode, "Community within a Community," p. 196.

prestige accorded them by the public not only must they not exploit these opportunities, but the public must not interpret as exploitation what the profession views as a proper relationship with clients.

The medical profession partakes in some degree of all these characteristics of a profession. The medical recruit must undergo a long period of training. After successfully surmounting the educational hurdle he may be admitted to the professional body and licensed to practise medicine. In his professional role he is expected to follow the ethics prescribed for his professional behaviour; he must maintain a required standard of technical competence in practice and remain subject to the discipline of his professional body. But a physician is also unlike most other professionals. He is expected to be emotionally neutral during his treatment of patients; he has access to a patient's body which would be allowed to no other person; he is privy to the intimate details of the lives of patients; he has contact with their suffering and death. His role is made even more demanding because he must deal with bodily functions which the layman considers aesthetically unattractive and because of his knowledge that in much of what he attempts a great deal of uncertainty as to outcome prevails.

Within these general features of the physician's role certain variations are evident. The degree of specialization is a crucial determinant of role variation in medicine. As medical knowledge grows, new specialties emerge or old ones divide into sub-specialties. The profession of medicine thus becomes an amalgamation of specialists and general practitioners with varying degrees of prestige attached to them. Since their training, tasks, and goals differ, specialists will differ in interests, and in the organization of their activities, but the strength of the medical culture as a whole enables the profession to limit the effects of these differences. Furthermore, specialization generates interdependence of specialists within the profession such that the individual practitioner is dependent upon other specialist colleagues for consultation and advice, for treatment facilities, for professional advancement and income. From this dependence flows a professional solidarity, a mutual reinforcement of each other's point of view on their rights, duties, and obligations.

THE PATIENT'S ROLE

Every social role is at least two sided and the investigator cannot understand one side without examining the other. To understand the role of the physician requires an understanding of the role of the patient. To the latter we now turn and first to its general features followed by examples of the manner in which social factors generate variations in that role.

To say that there is a social role for the sick person is another way of saying that certain social expectations prevail to which a patient must conform if those who seek to treat and care for him are to discharge their responsibilities effectively. Society expects a patient to act in a certain way and these expectations constrain his behaviour as a patient. Once he has been defined as a patient, society exempts the individual from his normal social responsibilities and at the same time it recognizes that he is not to blame for his condition. On the other hand, society expects that the patient will want to regain his health by seeking the services of those technically competent to provide them.[9] Variations in the performance of the role of patient may, however, occur as a result of psychological and cultural factors. King points out, for example, that the desire to regain health may not always be strong:

The enforced state of dependency in illness can gratify strong needs to be taken care of, as the individual was cared for as a child. Freedom from ordinary social responsibility can be a joy to some people, a state not to be surrendered easily. Hospital staff members are familiar with the patient who has a resurgence of symptoms sometimes of sufficient severity as to require continued hospitalization. Staff are also familiar with the malingerer who may feign illness or magnify his symptoms beyond demonstrable severity in order to be placed in the sick role, or who may wish to stay in the hospital beyond the time when medical decision seeks his discharge.[10]

Such cultural factors in variations in the sick role become important in relation to who defines illness as such. The layman's conception of disease obviously will differ from that of the physician, and among laymen there will be substantial divergence of views concerning the definition of illness. In his 1954 study of a small town in New York State, the late Professor Koos showed significant differences in the definition of illness among different social groups. He divided the study population into three classes, the major criteria of class being the occupation of the head of the family. Class I consisted of family heads who were business or professional men; Class II consisted of skilled or semi-skilled workers and farmers; Class III included labourers. The class distribution of the study population was as follows: Class I, 10 per cent; Class II, 65 per cent; Class III, 25 per cent. There was substantial variation between classes in the definition of what symptoms constituted illness. Table 1 shows the results when respondents were given a list of seventeen symptoms and asked to indicate which would require the attention of a physician. An awareness of the signifi-

9 / Stanley H. King, "Social Psychological Factors in Illness," in Howard E. Freeman *et al.* (eds.), *Handbook of Medical Sociology*, Englewood Cliffs, N.J.: Prentice-Hall, Inc., 1963, p. 112.
10 / *Ibid.*, pp. 112–13.

TABLE 1
Percentage of Respondents in Each Social Class Recognizing Specified
Symptoms as Needing Medical Attention*

Symptom	Class I (N = 51)	Class II (N = 335)	Class III (N = 128)
Loss of appetite	57	50	20
Persistent backache	53	44	19
Continued coughing	77	78	23
Persistent joint and muscle pains	80	47	19
Blood in stool	98	89	60
Blood in urine	100	93	69
Excessive vaginal bleeding	92	83	54
Swelling of ankles	77	76	23
Loss of weight	80	51	21
Bleeding gums	79	51	20
Chronic fatigue	80	53	19
Shortness of breath	77	55	21
Persistent headaches	80	56	22
Fainting spells	80	51	33
Pain in chest	80	51	31
Lump in breast	94	71	44
Lump in abdomen	92	65	34

*Percentages rounded to nearest whole number.
SOURCE: E. L. Koos, *The Health of Regionville*, New York:
Columbia University Press, 1954, p. 32.

cance of all these symptoms was uniformly high among all Class I respondents; Class II showed less sensitivity; Class III showed a general indifference to most symptoms.

Zborowski has shown that cultural factors affect the sick role.[11] In a study of three cultural groups, Jewish, Italian, and "Old American," he found that members of the three groups reacted differently to pain. The Jewish sufferer reacted by creating worry and concern in his group concerning his health, whereas the Italian attempted to gain sympathy for his suffering. In the first case the reaction to pain tended to generate the support of the family and the physician which was directed towards a complete cure; the Italian reaction tended to generate efforts to relieve the pain. The "Old American" attitude towards pain differed from the other two in that while the individual was disturbed by the clinical implications of the pain and was worried about its restrictive effect on his activities, he was optimistic about the results of the application of science and skill in his case.

11 / Mark Zborowski, "Cultural Components in Response to Pain," *Journal of Social Issues*, no. 8, 1952, pp. 16–30.

These examples provide some indication of the manner in which psychological, social, and cultural factors can create variations in the performance of the patient's role such that his expectations do not coincide with those of the physician.

A relatively simple model of the interaction between two individuals serves as a convenient first step in an analysis of the concept of role strain. In the interaction between two people the behaviour of each tends to conform to the expectations of the other, but this result is not without its cost because the expectations of the one partner may serve to limit and restrict the behaviour of the other, and thereby induce strain in both. Reciprocal knowledge of each other's expectations stems from the values that each has learned during socialization. An individual learns that conformity to these values brings reward and gratification and that non-conformity results in deprivation and punishment. Individuals seek to maximize gratifications and minimize deprivations and this attempt leads to a desire to conform. The expectations which one person lives up to are not gratifications in themselves but by conforming to them he thereby gains rewards in the form of approval and esteem of others.

The failure of one individual to meet the expectations of the other introduces a strain into the relationship. The interaction between physician and patient, for example, requires behaviour considered appropriate for each in that situation. For easy performance of each role there would be a required pattern of behaviour which is known to both the incumbent and to those who interact with him. The expectations of each provide a framework for action between them, and if the price of this interaction is to be minimized these expectations must remain in balance; they must fit together so that the interaction based on them can proceed in a predictable manner. To the extent that there is imbalance, and the actions of the other cannot be foreseen, the result will be anxiety and strain.

The lack of balance of expectations so far as professional and client are concerned may stem from conditions in the social system such as the situation in which the professional work is carried on. Again, the expectations may be so detailed and involved that the individual cannot comprehend them. On the other hand, they may be vague and lack sufficient detail so that the individual has no clear conception of what is expected of him. One last source of strain stems from the contradictory character of some expectations. All of these conditions introduce disturbances in the balance of expectations, and thereby place a strain on the individual.

Any individual has a number of roles; the physician, for example, besides his professional role may have a role as father, husband, brother, administrator, and so on. Any situation calls for those involved to act in a manner prescribed by their particular role in that situation.

It is within this structure of a number of roles that further strains are located. Individuals interact in a variety of patterned ways, and it is these patterns which the sociologist must examine in order to determine the social genesis of behaviour, not forgetting, of course, that individuals with a variety of personality idiosyncrasies can occupy the same role. The social structure may impose strains, but these are reflected on different personalities. The latter are the result of biological endowment and past experience during childhood when personality characteristics are moulded. In a sense then, personalities must be fitted to roles, and in the interplay between the two a lack of fit may impose varying degrees of strain on the individual.

The integration of personality and role may involve strain *within* the role. This can be seen, for example, in the situation in which expectations have been insufficiently "embedded" in the personality so that the appropriate stimulus does not "set them up," and the individual has difficulty in fulfilling his role obligations. There is another possibility, that of the conflict *between* roles. In this case, the individual is faced with divergent expectations in different roles. The physician, for example, may fulfil the requirements of that role in his office, in the hospital, or in the patient's home, but he must put that role aside when he goes home to wife and children. In the latter situation he faces a set of expectations which differ from those he faces in his professional role.

The degree of strain imposed upon the individual as he goes about attempting to fulfil the obligations of a succession of roles varies with their degree of incompatibility. In any case, conflict of roles is an endemic feature of social life; it is a reflection of the fact that no society is perfectly integrated, in the sense that it allows for no inconsistencies in or between the content of its structure of roles. It is exposure to this type of malintegration within the social structure which leads to strain. When the social structure is changing at a rapid pace the possibility of malintegration and consequent strain is greatly increased.

A further possibility of strain stems from the fact that in the performance of any one role the individual interacts with a number of others who occupy a range of different roles. The physician, for example, in his role as physician maintains relationships with patients, patients' families, hospital administrators, nurses, paramedical personnel, other physicians, and third parties such as officials of medical care insurance plans and government. Individuals in these different roles may have divergent expectations and obligations. In an era of rapid social change when medical knowledge is expanding at an increasing rate, and when a shortage of physicians and a more highly educated and medically sophisticated public make severe and sometimes impossible demands on the time, energy, and skill of the practitioner, he faces severe strain. These demands are particularly exacting when the commitment to an accepted manner of practising restricts the ability of the physician to attempt to alleviate these strains with different ways of organizing practice which could reduce the demands upon him.[12]

THE FUNCTION OF IDEOLOGY

A most important characteristic of any professional group is its professional culture: its values, norms, and symbols. Values embrace those fundamental beliefs of the profession upon which its continued existence is claimed to rest.

Foremost among these values is the essential worth of the services which the professional group extends to the community. The profession considers that the service is a social good and that community welfare would be immeasurably impaired by its absence. The twin concepts of professional authority and monopoly also possess the force of group value. Thus, the proposition that in all service related matters the professional group is infinitely wiser than the laity is regarded as beyond argument. Likewise non-arguable is the proposition that acquisition by the professional group of a service monopoly would inevitably produce social progress. And then there is the value of rationality; that is, the commitment to objectivity in the realm of theory and technique. By virtue of this orientation, nothing of a theoretical or technical nature is regarded as sacred and unchallengeable simply because it has a history of acceptance and use.[13]

A professional ideology consisting of a set of ideas, values, and beliefs concerning the nature of the professional role, its relationship to other social roles, and to the society, attempts to resolve the conflicting demands and strains facing the professional in a changing society. The medical ideology differs from that of the business man, the engineer, the lawyer, and members of other professions since the physician faces different sets of problems. Not all the elements of an ideology are peculiar to the profes-

12 / For a theoretical discussion of ways in which a profession may reduce role strain for its members see Goode, "Community within a Community," pp. 196–97.

13 / Ernest Greenwood, "Attributes of a Profession," *Social Work*, vol. 2, no. 3, July 1957, as quoted by Howard M. Vollmer and Donald L. Mills, eds., *Professionalization*, Englewood Cliffs, N.J.: Prentice-Hall, Inc., 1966, pp. 16–17.

sion which uses them; some are generally accepted social values, more widely distributed throughout the society,[14] which provide the ideological framework within which the particular professional ideology must be expressed. Humanitarianism, for example, while being a central idea in the practice of medicine, is not the prerogative of that profession only. Ideas about the particular nature of the doctor-patient relationship, on the other hand, are peculiar to medicine. The ideology of the medical profession is thus linked to the general cultural tradition of our society. The physician's commitment to this ideology, while it enables him to meet, in part at least, the strains which he encounters in his professional capacity, also makes his ideological reaction to his problem socially acceptable.

When a profession faces change or when it is under attack, it will emphasize its beliefs as a means of defending itself. "Where a role involves patterns of conflicting demands, the occupants of that role may respond by elaborating a system of ideas and symbols, which in part may serve as a guide to action, but chiefly has broader and more direct functions as a response to strain."[15]

Like other professions which serve clients, the medical profession faces a changing world in which the conflicting demands of those whom they serve, and with whom they serve, impose severe pressures upon the practitioner. In what situations do these pressures occur? The following chapters attempt to answer this question.

14 / Vernon K. Dibble, "Occupations and Ideologies," *American Journal of Sociology*, vol. 67, no. 2, September 1962, pp. 229–30.

15 / Francis X. Sutton *et al.*, *The American Business Creed*, Cambridge, Mass.: Harvard University Press, 1956, p. 308.

3

MEDICAL EDUCATION

IT IS WITHIN the medical school that the aspiring physician receives most if not all of his formal medical education. As he goes through this stage in his professional preparation, the school will provide him with professional knowledge and skills, and "a professional identity so that he comes to think, act, and feel like a physician."[1] It is the school's "problem to enable the medical man to live up to the expectations of the professional role long after he has left the sustaining value-environment provided by the medical school."[2]

The organization and content of medical education today are under critical scrutiny to determine if the educational process can produce physicians competent to meet the new and old problems facing the practitioner in a changing society. Although they must still provide practitioners qualified to treat human ills, medical educators are asking whether the various types of physicians they train have, in fact, acquired the knowledge and skills required to meet the health problems generated by a rapidly changing society. As illustrated in chapter 1 these problems include the growth of specialization; the changing nature of the health problems facing society as a result of the application of increased scientific knowledge; demographic change; the rise in incomes and the accompanying increase in the demand for medical care of the highest quality on the part of consumers with a greater degree of sophistication in health matters than previous generations and increasingly critical of the medical services they receive; and changing social values with an increasing emphasis on collective as opposed to individual action in attempts to solve the health problems of society and the resulting conception of medical care as a civic right. To cope with these problems the medical school today must endeavour to have among its graduates an ever more varied group:

1 / R. K. Merton, *et al.* (eds.), *The Student-Physician*, Cambridge, Mass.: Harvard University Press, 1957, p. 7.
2 / *Ibid.*

[It] must provide, somehow, generalists with a wide range of knowledge and skills; specialists with a profundity of insight and the capacity to manage increasingly intricate facilities; research men who can move medicine steadily forward toward new goals; medical men akin in function and in spirit to systems engineers – all of these in greater numbers than ever before: and it must do all this in the face of an insatiable public demand for accomplishment. Nothing of this sort has ever before been asked of an educational establishment.[3]

The contemporary critical scrutiny of medical education is not the first. The Flexner Report in 1910 was the culmination of a period of criticism of medical education in both the United States and Canada which resulted in its transformation from an apprenticeship system, under which the student gained his professional knowledge while working with a medical practitioner, to a recognized discipline within a university.[4] Flexner made these observations about medical education in Canada:

In the matter of medical schools, Canada reproduces the United States on a greatly reduced scale. Western University (London) is as bad as anything to be found on this side of the line; Laval and Halifax Medical College are feeble; Winnipeg and Kingston represent a distinct effort toward higher ideals; McGill and Toronto are excellent. The eight schools of the Dominion thus belong to three different types, the best adding a fifth year to their advantages of superior equipment and instruction.[5]

The weaknesses in medical education noted by Flexner in the United States culminated in the closing of a number of medical schools, the so-called "diploma mills," and the building of new and the strengthening of existing schools both of which were closely integrated with university communities through the appointment of full-time clinical teachers. Similar developments, although at a slower pace, occurred in Canada.

In spite of the present pressures upon it medical education today, to a large extent, remains cast in the mould prescribed by Flexner, but because of them the student's image of himself as a physician has more unknowns and is more obscure than in any previous era. For example, the strengthening of the professional education of the physician, in terms of content and quality, as a result of Flexner's recommendations tended to overlook the increasing degree of specialization within medicine due to the growing

3 / Oliver Cope and Jerrold Zacharias, *Medical Education Reconsidered*, Philadelphia: J. B. Lippincott Co., 1966, pp. 23–24.
4 / Abraham Flexner, *Medical Education in the United States and Canada*, A Report to the Carnegie Foundation for the Advancement of Teaching, Bulletin no. 4, New York: 1910.   5 / *Ibid.*, p. 325.

body of medical knowledge. Today no individual physician can encompass it, "yet, to a large extent, the medical school continues to operate on the assumption that he must. As a consequence the medical student faces the unbearable task of seeking to master an overwhelming range of knowledge and skills that he may never utilize in his career – a fact of which he is well aware even as a student."[6]

Since these pressures, and possibly others yet to emerge, are not likely to lessen their impact on medical education and on the organization and content of medical care, the crucial problem for the medical student and the practitioner is the manner in which he is to adjust to a changing medical and social world. In such a world adjustment is never complete. As Hughes points out,

Some will doubtless accept the implications of open-endedness more than others; some may indeed make it part of their identity to be men who do not seek a fixed identity, men whose constant is that they are open to change, or even men who seek the spots where change is the major assignment. Others may seek, successfully or not, the spots which appear most fixed, the bastions that appear safe from storming.[7]

ORGANIZATIONAL PRESSURES

In Canada each medical school or faculty is an integral part of a university. It is headed by a dean who is appointed by the board of governors of the university on the advice of its president. The school is divided into departments each of which is the responsibility of a department head. Department heads and senior faculty are usually selected by departmental committees chaired by the dean but the actual appointment must be approved by the university board of governors. Junior faculty are usually selected by the department head and the members of that department. In most cases the dean leaves the responsibility for such appointments with the departments, but he must recommend them to the president who then places them before the board of governors for formal approval.

As knowledge expands and specialties proliferate the number of departments increases, which can intensify competition for the available teaching resources such as curriculum time, equipment, and beds in the teaching hospital. This competition is accompanied by a demand for an increasing degree of departmental autonomy with the result that some departments will be relatively isolated and have only a limited conception of what is

6 / *Ibid.*, p. 34.
7 / Everett C. Hughes, "The Making of a Physician," *Human Organization*, vol. 14, no. 4, 1956, p. 25.

being taught in others. Such isolation may be particularly apparent between two types of departments, the clinical departments and the basic science departments. The clinical departments, such as medicine, surgery, obstetrics and gynaecology, psychiatry, and paediatrics, are usually based in the teaching hospital and staffed in the main, or until recently, entirely by physicians whose primary role has been the practice of their specialty. The basic science departments, such as anatomy, biochemistry, pharmacology, physiology, pathology, and bacteriology, are based in the medical school and are usually staffed by basic scientists whose primary role is teaching and research. The isolation between these two main divisions of clinical and basic science departments is strengthened by the demands of basic scientists for autonomy and status as scientists which they see as resulting from the integration of their scientific activities with those in corresponding departments of the university outside the medical school.

These demands of the basic scientists are based in part on their claims of greater economy and efficiency in the operation of one rather than two departments in the same discipline, one in the medical school and one in the university at large, and in part on their realization that because their teaching and research activities are focussed on the field of medicine rather than on their particular fields of science, they are open to control by teaching physicians. This control is resented by some basic scientists who feel that the teaching physicians do not understand their scientific orientation. MacFarlane shows the extent to which basic science departments in 1961–62 were staffed by basic scientists without an MD degree (Table 2).

TABLE 2
Percentage of Teachers of Basic Science of Rank of Assistant Professor or Higher in Twelve Canadian Medical Schools by Subject, 1961–62

Subject	M.D. Total	PH.D. (D.PHIL., D.SC.) Total	M.D. and PH.D. Total	No doctoral degree Total
Anatomy	55	19	21	5
Physiology	45.5	41.5	12	1
Biochemistry	8	83	6.6	2.4
Pharmacology	33	50	12.5	4.5
Microbiology	55	27	12	6
Pathology	74	10	13	3

SOURCE: J. A. MacFarlane, *Medical Education in Canada*, Royal Commission on Health Services, Ottawa: Queen's Printer, 1964, p. 133.

The departments of biochemistry, pharmacology, and physiology are particularly noticeable for the high proportion of faculty who do not possess medical qualifications.

The degree of commitment of medical faculty to their teaching role, as reflected in the type of appointment, creates a further division in the medical school. Appointments in basic science departments are on a regular full-time basis, but those in clinical departments are of three types: full-time, geographic full-time, and part-time. The full-time teacher is one whose sole source of remuneration is the university. The geographic full-time teacher is primarily responsible to the medical school from which he receives at least one-half of his income; he may, however, treat his own patients in the teaching hospital affiliated with the medical school, but there may be limits on the amount he may earn in this way, and on the amount of time he may devote to this activity. The part-time teacher is a practising physician who devotes a limited amount of time to teaching. Since the part-time clinical teachers also have a full-time independent practice they are less committed to a teaching career than their full-time teaching colleagues in both basic science and clinical departments. Their monetary rewards for teaching are usually minimal, but other rewards in the form of professional prestige and a consequent ability to attract patients and attain consultant status for their non-teaching practising colleagues may be enhanced, thus increasing their earning power to substantially more than that of their full-time teaching colleagues. On the other hand, it is the full-time and geographic full-time teachers whose contributions to the advancement of medical knowledge through research provide the basis for their own reputation and that of the medical school. In a sense, the part-time teacher gains prestige from his association with a medical school to whose reputation he may contribute very little because of his greater commitment to a full-time practice. This situation may create difficulties in the relationship between full- and part-time teachers. These will not be eased by a realization on the part of the former that the medical school could not operate without the services of low-paid part-time teachers and avoid substantial increases in costs. For example, in the academic year 1961–62, in the then existing twelve Canadian medical schools nearly 88 per cent of all teachers were part-time.[8]

The medical school curriculum, now under critical examination by medical educators, for the most part changes slowly although much of the recently discovered subject-matter can no longer be taught to students in terms of the traditional medical or pre-medical curriculum organization. In his first year at a traditional medical school, the student will be exposed to anatomy, histology, genetics, biochemistry, human physiology, and a varying amount of social or behavioural science. In the second year he will

8 / J. A. MacFarlane, *Medical Education in Canada*, Royal Commission on Health Services, Ottawa: Queen's Printer, 1964, p. 95.

take courses in pharmacology, microbiology, pathology, and neuro-anatomy and will learn more about the significance of the basic medical sciences for the clinical aspects of medicine. During first and second years he is exposed to patients through bedside and classroom demonstrations and in second year he becomes familiar with methods of interviewing and physical examination. In his last two years of medical school the student comes into increasing contact with patients. In this he is supervised by teachers in the departments of surgery, medicine, obstetrics, gynaecology, paediatrics, psychiatry and possibly others. In his final year, as a clinical clerk, he becomes a more or less essential member of the hospital's care team, more and more performing the duties of the intern for a limited number of patients.

Kendall's findings concerning changes in the curriculum would suggest that if change threatens departmental autonomy, the pace of change is likely to be slow if not imperceptible, and that despite their claims that changes are necessary in the medical school curriculum, medical educators tend "*as a whole*, not to recommend any changes at all."[9] This tendency is particularly obvious in the older basic science courses.[10]

The teaching methods, as distinct from the curriculum, in the medical school are varied. They include supervised practical work on the wards, demonstrations in the surgical theatre of the teaching hospital, case conferences, laboratory exercises in chemical pathology, and lectures in public health, social medicine, environmental medicine, ethics, the history of medicine, and health economics. MacFarlane has criticized this system of teaching because it treats the student more as a high school student than a mature university student who is capable of assuming greater responsibilities than he is given.[11]

Emerging trends in the medical curriculum and in teaching methods may offset the organizational pressures facing the medical school and the difficulties they create for the medical student. Macleod claims that present research in medical education seeks to determine "whether the curriculum fits the objectives and to evaluate impersonally the procedures used and the quality of the product."[12] In Canada, however, innovations in medical education have been accepted slowly. To illustrate this point he quotes the comment made by joint American-Canadian survey teams after their periodic visits to Canadian medical schools.

9 / Patricia L. Kendall, "Clinical Teachers' Views of the Basic Science Curriculum," *Journal of Medical Education*, vol. 35, no. 2, February 1960, p. 157.

10 / *Ibid.*

11 / MacFarlane, *Medical Education in Canada*, p. 80.

12 / J. Wendell Macleod, "Curriculum in Canadian Medical Education," *Canadian Medical Association Journal*, vol. 88, April 6, 1963, pp. 705–12.

Compared with many medical schools on this continent yours [the Canadian medical school] depends on relatively more formal didactic teaching; it gives many more lectures and its laboratory courses are more rigidly standardized. In most departments your teachers attempt more complete coverage of subject matter. Students are given less clinical responsibility and are given it later than in many other schools.[13]

This illustration indicates the conservative bias of medical education in Canada, which is manifested in the "cultural lag" in the implementation of educational innovations introduced elsewhere, particularly in the United States.

Having satisfactorily completed the four years of instruction as determined by examinations at the end of each academic year, the medical student is granted the MD degree, but permission to practise does not automatically follow the award of this degree. The licence to practise in any particular province is granted only after the student has met the requirements of the provincial College of Physicians and Surgeons, the body which has the statutory authority to grant such a license. However, before the student is granted this right he must serve an internship of one year's duration in a hospital approved for that purpose by the College. In one medical school the final examination for the degree is deferred until completion of the internship with the medical school designating those hospitals in which the intern year may be served.

From the foregoing it is obvious that an integral element in a medical education programme is a teaching hospital. Although as yet no medical school in Canada owns and operates its own university hospital a number are either being built or are in various stages of planning. The prevailing arrangement is for a medical school to enter into a contractual agreement with an accredited hospital for the use of part of its facilities for the treatment of patients who become the responsibility of the medical school teaching staff. Before the introduction of hospital insurance in Canada these university-affiliated hospitals had substantial numbers of charity patients. Although these patients could not afford the costs of medical care the medical school teaching staff provided them with a high quality of care. For their part these patients agreed to being used as teaching material.

A number of difficulties may arise in the relationship between the medical school and the university-affiliated teaching hospital. These may derive, in part, from their seemingly divergent goals. On the one hand, the medical school is primarily interested in teaching and research; on the other the teaching hospital focusses its attention on patient care and com-

13 / *Ibid.*, p. 6.

munity service. The possibilities of conflict between these two sets of goals are obvious. Difficulties may also emerge in appointments to the teaching staff of the hospital. Such appointments are the responsibility of the medical school, and not the least of the rewards of such an appointment is the prestige and professional standing that it gives to the appointee. That the control over such appointments should create some difficulty between medical schools and the medical authority of the teaching hospital is not surprising. Other difficulties may result from attempts by the medical school on the one hand, and the non-faculty medical staff of the teaching hospital on the other, to control the work of interns and residents who may be a major source of assistance in the hospital practice of the latter. The responsibility for patients admitted to the teaching unit, the possibility of different standards of patient care in the hospital and in its teaching unit, and the conduct of research in the teaching unit may be additional sources of difficulty in the relationship between the medical school and the teaching hospital.[14]

THE MEDICAL SCHOOL AND THE MEDICAL STUDENT

We have mentioned that the medical school provides the student with professional knowledge and skills and a professional identity so that when he enters practice he will think, act, and feel like a physician. This process of moulding the student to a pre-existing pattern is termed socialization by sociologists; the mould is determined by the groups to which the individual belongs and their effect on him is the result of his interaction with other members of these groups. In the medical school the medical student interacts with faculty members and other medical students primarily, but also with others such as nurses and a range of paramedical personnel. "Since the patterns of social interaction of medical students with these others are only similar and not identical, the variations result in different kinds of medical men emerging from what may at first seem to be the 'same' social environment of the medical school."[15] It is this structure of social relationships of which he is a part that operates to produce strain and anxiety for the medical student, and so can affect the extent to which he assimilates the established medical culture.

The effect of these strains and the consequent anxiety depends to some extent on the social background of the medical student. Persons with a similar cultural background will tend to react to strain in a similar manner. Data on the social background of Canadian medical students are very

14 / MacFarlane, *Medical Education in Canada*, pp. 114–16.
15 / Merton *et al.*, *The Student-Physician*, p. 287.

TABLE 3
Percentage Distribution of Active Civilian Physicians by Father's Occupational Class
at Time of Entering University by the Type of Work, Canada, 1962 (N = 9,848)

Father's occupational class	Type of work				1961 labour force
	General practitioners	Specialists*	Other†	Total	
I	25.9	32.3	31.2	29.9	3.9
II	4.3	4.2	4.6	4.4	4.3
III	38.5	39.6	38.0	38.8	9.0
IV	9.9	9.0	10.1	9.6	19.8
V	11.4	8.6	9.4	9.7	32.2
VI	10.0	6.3	6.7	7.6	30.8
Total	100.0	100.0	100.0	100.0	100.0

*"Specialists" includes specialists, consultants, research and teaching, public health, and industrial medicine.
†"Other" includes interns, residents, fellows, hospital staff, medical assessment, medical directors, others.
SOURCE: Royal Commission on Health Services, Survey of Physicians in Canada, 1962.

limited[16] but some data are available for former students who were practising physicians in 1962. In the survey of physicians undertaken by the Royal Commission on Health Services in that year, each respondent was asked to state his father's occupation at the time the respondent entered university. These occupational data were arranged in six occupational classes according to the weight given to each occupation's socio-economic index based on the education, income, and prestige of the occupation.[17] The data, contained in Table 3, show that a disproportionate share of Canadian physicians, not quite 30 per cent, are drawn from the highest class, as compared with almost 4 per cent representation of the 1961

16 / D. G. Fish and G. G. Clarke, "Medical Students in Canadian Universities," *Canadian Medical Association Journal*, vol. 94, April 2, 1966, pp. 693–700. The Association of Canadian Medical Colleges maintains a statistical record of medical students enrolled in Canadian medical schools, but its data show only enrolment trends, withdrawals, dismissals, citizenship, geographic origin, place of permanent residence, and other characteristics. These statistics show that enrolment for the academic years 1957–58 to 1965–66 rose from 3,683 to 4,023; that during this period the percentage of women medical students rose from 7.0 to 11.4; that in 1965–66 just over 89 per cent of medical students were Canadian citizens; and that in 1965–66 with the exception of medical schools at McGill and Queen's universities, over 90 per cent of medical students were attending medical schools in their province of permanent residence.
17 / For a description of the method used in the construction of this index see: Bernard R. Blishen, "A Socio-Economic Index for Occupations in Canada," *Canadian Review of Sociology and Anthropology*, vol. 4, no. 1, 1967, pp. 41–53.

Canadian labour force in the same class. No matter what the type of work in which they are engaged, general practice, specialty practice, or some other form of practice, the disproportionate representation of physicians in the highest class is evident. In fact, over 73 per cent of the physicians had fathers who were members of the three top classes and only just over 17 per cent of the 1961 labour force were represented in these same classes.

Since social classes develop class sub-cultures, and each sub-culture develops its own distinctive values, styles of life, life goals, and rules of behaviour, it is evident that a substantial proportion of Canadian medical students have a relatively homogeneous social background that will be reflected in the behaviour, attitudes, values, and aspirations they bring with them as they enter medical school.

The tendency for physicians to be recruited from the upper social levels of society is also evident when the occupational background of the fathers of medical students is examined. Table 4 indicates the occupation of the fathers of general practitioners and specialists practising in Canada in 1962, the time these physicians entered university. The data refer only to

TABLE 4
Percentage Distribution for Canada of General Practitioners and Specialists by Occupational Group of Father at Time of Entering University, 1962

Occupational group	General practitioners	Specialists	Labour force 15 years of age and over* 1951	1961
1. Managerial, professional	54.4	65.8	14.3	18.3
2. Clerical, sales, service and recreation	12.4	11.9	18.1	21.6
3. Transportation, communication	3.7	2.7	9.3	7.7
4. Craftsmen, production process	9.9	8.4	25.3	29.6
5. Farmers, farm workers	16.4	8.7	19.6	12.5
6. Loggers, fishermen, miners	0.9	0.9	5.3	3.9
7. Labourers	2.3	1.5	8.1	6.4
Total	100.0	99.9	100.0	100.0

*Excludes "Occupation not stated."
SOURCE: Royal Commission on Health Services, *Survey of Physicians in Canada*, 1962.

physicians in non-administrative positions, that is, they exclude physicians holding positions such as hospital administrator.[18]

This table shows clearly that in Canada both general practitioners and specialists tend to come from families in which the father has a managerial or professional occupation. This tendency is particularly evident in the case of specialists. When comparing the occupational distribution of the fathers of present-day physicians with that of the total labour force it is evident that the managerial and professional occupations are over represented. All other occupations are under represented.

The tendency for medical students to be drawn disproportionately from families in which the father has a professional or managerial occupational role is evident in both Canada and the United States. Judek's figure of 56.2 per cent[19] can be compared with the 58 per cent reported for a study undertaken by Gee in 1956 in the United States.[20]

The degree of occupational inheritance in medicine, i.e., the tendency for sons to follow the same occupation as their fathers, is shown by data derived from the survey of physicians undertaken by the Royal Commission on Health Services referred to above. These data indicate that in 1962 just over 15 per cent of Canadian-born physicians had fathers, living or dead, who were physicians. This is somewhat higher than the 11 per cent reported by Gee.[21]

These data on the social background of Canadian medical students provide some indication of the social pre-conditioning which may sustain the medical student as he attempts to cope with the strains and anxieties engendered by the process of medical education. They also provide evidence to support Hall's claim that the ambition to study medicine is largely social in nature; it is generated in and nourished by the groups to which the student belongs.[22] Evidently, for 15 per cent of former Canadian medical students their ambition to become physicians was generated within the family in which the financial resources to support the ambition were available and in which the role model of the father was a continuing example of

18 / Since we are examining the occupational background of the father of the physician at the time the physician first entered university, the correct procedure would be to provide occupational groups prevailing at the time the physician first entered university. In the case of the older physicians this may go back a number of decades prior to the latest list of occupational groups published by the Dominion Bureau of Statistics in 1961.

19 / S. Judek, *Medical Manpower in Canada*, Royal Commission on Health Services, Ottawa: Queen's Printer, 1964, p. 11.

20 / Helen Hofer Gee, "The Student View of the Medical Admission Process," *Journal of Medical Education*, vol. 32, no. 10, October 1957, part 2, p. 143.

21 / *Ibid.*

22 / Oswald Hall, "The Stages of a Medical Career," *American Journal of Sociology*, vol. 53, March 1948, pp. 327–36.

what the future held. For another 41 per cent the family provided the financial means to support the ambition.

Despite this similarity in the social background of a high proportion of medical students, the cross pressures evident in the organization of the medical school and its affiliated teaching hospital, can, as noted above, have consequences for their socialization and subsequent careers as practising physicians.

These organizational pressures in the medical school serve to confuse the student as to the appropriate values applicable to the practical exigencies of situations in the school but particularly in practice. Even without these stresses the student faces the problem of acquiring values and norms which are seemingly incompatible. Merton claims that "for each norm there tends to be at least one coordinate norm, which is, if not inconsistent with the other, at least sufficiently different as to make it difficult for the student and the physician to live up to them both.... From this perspective, medical education can be conceived as facing the task of enabling students to learn *how to blend* incompatible or potentially incompatible norms into a functionally consistent whole." For example, "the physician must be emotionally detached in his attitudes toward patients, keeping 'his emotions on ice' and not becoming 'overly identified' with his patients. *But*: he must avoid becoming callous through excessive detachment, and should have compassionate concern for the patient."[23] Unless the student can find some way of effectively meeting these strains as they emerge in his day-to-day experience his transition from student to physician will be difficult. The degree of difficulty he faces will depend to a large extent on the degree to which he can divest himself of some of the values he holds when he enters medicine, and on his learning the values of the medical student culture which will enable him to face the pressures produced by the organization of the medical school.

Becker and Geer claim that the social organization of the medical school creates pressures upon the students such that the idealism with which they entered medicine, although never lost, is displaced by a protective veneer of cynicism as they progress through this stage of their careers. They are told that they cannot learn all that there is to know in medicine, they therefore become selective in what they learn based on their ideas about the nature of future practice and on what they think their teachers consider of sufficient importance to be asked in examinations. These ideas become part of the student culture, based upon the student's day-to-day experience in the medical school, with its own values and modes of behaviour which obscure the initial idealism but support

23 / Merton *et al.*, *The Student-Physician*, pp. 72–74.

him as he attempts to cope with the situations he meets. As his contacts with patients increase, the student becomes increasingly concerned with the technical details of therapy and views the patient in terms of the problems he poses for which the student must find an answer. As graduation approaches, this student culture is gradually displaced by the original idealism.[24] This idealism cannot sustain the individual as he seeks to master day-to-day contingencies; it is therefore pushed aside to be replaced by values applicable to immediate situations. It reappears, as the possibility of professional practice becomes more immediate, "but it now has a more specific character, consisting of concrete ideas about how certain problems of medical practice are to be faced."[25]

There can be little doubt that the organizational pressures evident in the medical school have an effect on the socialization of the medical student. This effect is evident not only in the manner in which he learns to deal with incompatible values, but also in his attempt to master the curriculum, in his choice of a type of practice, and in his reaction to the demands of internship and residency.

The growing corpus of medical knowledge and its fragmentation into numerous medical and scientific specialties within the medical school pose pressing problems concerning the manner in which this expanding body of material can be effectively taught to the medical student so that he comprehends the fragments as part of an integrated whole. This development is accompanied by the growing importance of the teaching hospital where the equipment, the paramedical personnel, and patients are located. Acting as an apprentice under the guidance of his teachers the medical student learns his craft within this type of institution. But the teaching hospitals are staffed by highly specialized physicians who focus their skills "upon major illness, the problem case and highly technical investigation."[26] This focus imparts a distorted perspective to the student whose case load when he enters practice may embrace more than the major acute illnesses he studies in the teaching hospital, and may require something less than the highly technical facilities and services available there.

The crucial problem for the medical educator is to integrate the advances in medicine in such a way that the medical student can apply them when he enters practice. In his attempts to solve this problem he faces a particularly difficult obstacle. If the student is to be taught as much of the

24 / Howard S. Becker and Blanche Geer, "The Fate of Idealism in Medical School," *American Sociological Review*, vol. 23, February 1958, pp. 50–56.
25 / Howard S. Becker *et al.*, *Boys in White*, Chicago: University of Chicago Press, 1961, p. 430.
26 / MacFarlane, *Medical Education in Canada*, p. 33.

new, and old, medical knowledge and techniques as he requires to practise effectively more time is required to teach them. But the curriculum of the medical school is timebound; it cannot be expanded indefinitely. In fact, it can only be expanded within narrow limits. As Merton points out:

This means ... that departments and faculty members of the medical school in effect compete for the scarce time of the student just as patients compete for the scarce time of the physician. Hours of instruction are carefully computed and parceled out. The introduction of new teaching materials and courses must often be at the expense of other materials and courses.[27]

The medical student must not only try to synthesize the knowledge imparted to him into an integrated whole so that he is aware of the relationship between the various segments of the corpus of medical knowledge, but he must, if he is to be a successful student, pass the required examinations in the various basic science and clinical fields. Since success in these terms is the criterion by which he is judged by his teachers, the student concentrates his efforts on passing examinations. MacFarlane claims that "if one were to walk into a lecture room in the third year, he would hear an excellent outline of a particular aspect of medicine, and see the students urgently trying to commit to paper what the lecturer was saying, obviously for use at some future examination."[28]

The advance of medical knowledge and techniques, and the accompanying proliferation of specialists in the medical school and teaching hospital, as well as in medical practice, have resulted in a system of teaching which, as noted above, emphasizes particular problem cases of major illness requiring highly technical investigation. In his investigation of such cases the medical student loses sight of the person and his social environment which may have a substantial and direct bearing on his illness. With a less sophisticated system of medical knowledge, the physician could know most, if not all, that was required in a particular case, and still have sufficient time to understand at least the significant details of the patient's social background. As medical knowledge has increased, knowledge of the relationship between social factors and illness has remained almost undeveloped despite the fact that it was becoming increasingly important in the medical understanding of the patient and his illness. Thus the medical school now faces the problem of teaching medical students an integrated corpus of knowledge in the face of the growing specialization of medicine and the fragmentation of medical knowledge, and a complex

27 / Merton *et al.*, *The Student-Physician*, pp. 22–23.
28 / MacFarlane, *Medical Education in Canada*, p. 80.

social environment intimately connected with the genesis of illness. This problem is a crucial one for the medical educator for he knows that modern medicine is far more powerful than its predecessor, and that lack of knowledge, carelessness, or other faults of a practising physician can have dire consequences for his patients. Ellis describes this situation as follows:

The power of medicine to harm the patient has grown just as rapidly as its power to help. The physician and the general practitioner have joined the surgeon as people who by acts of commission and omission can do as much harm as good. Yet unlike him, and working in isolation under cramped conditions, and under pressure, seldom allowing for the quiet deliberate reflection which is needed, they can and are tempted to deploy powerful and dangerous remedies by a stroke of a fountain pen upon a prescription form....

The new medicine is more powerful, often more difficult, and usually much slower to practise than the old. It is consequently much more demanding of man-power and far more expensive.[29]

The increasing division of medical knowledge into specialties as reflected in the range of specialists represented in the medical school faculty also has an effect on the student's career interests. A study of medical students at the University of Kansas Medical School found that in their decision to take specialty training or training for general practice students used four main criteria. The most obvious of these was the time required to specialize which, depending upon the specialty, could take as long as five years. The second criterion used by the student was the spectrum of complaints he would be expected to treat in general as compared to specialty practice. He realized that he could not know all that there is to know about the range of ills he might be called upon to treat as a general practitioner. As a specialist, on the other hand, he could limit himself to a sector of knowledge and thereby know more about his chosen field. But if he restricted himself to a specialty he would miss the range of interesting cases requiring the services of the general practitioner. The third criterion was the student's conception of the amount of work demanded by each type of practice. Students saw the general practitioner as being under much more severe strain than the specialist because of the excessive demands for his services, demands over which he has little, if any, control. The fourth criterion was the extent to which a close personal relationship with patients can be maintained. Students saw the specialist as practising an impersonal technical type of medicine and the general practitioner as

29 / J. R. Ellis, "Tomorrow's Doctors," *British Medical Journal*, vol. 1, June 19, 1965, p. 1573.

TABLE 5
Interest of Canadian Medical Students in Various
Fields of Medical Practice

Field of medical practice	Percent of students selecting field as "1" in terms of interest	Over-all rank
General practice	26.6	1
Surgery	18.7	2
Internal medicine	18.5	3
Pediatrics	9.3	4
Psychiatry	9.1	5
Obstetrics	5.5	6
Research	3.7	7
Neurology	3.5	8
Medical teaching	2.3	9
Pathology	1.5	10
Dermatology	1.0	11
Administration	0.3	12

SOURCE: John H. Mount and D. G. Fish, "Canadian Medical Student Interest in General Practice and the Specialties," *Canadian Medical Association Journal*, vol. 94, April 2, 1966, pp. 2–6.

maintaining close and intimate contact with patients in the course of therapy.[30] In their choice of a particular specialty these students considered a number of factors. Among these were income, working hours, and amount of work, prestige of the specialty, the extent and type of relationship with patients, extent of medical responsibility, the extent to which medical knowledge in the specialty assures that the problems to be faced can be managed, and the length of the required residency.[31]

In a study undertaken in 1964 of a non-random sample of Canadian medical students, their interest in various fields of medical practice emerged as shown on Table 5. As the authors of this study are careful to point out, "if research, teaching and administration are excluded 67% of the medical students in this sample were more interested in a specialty than in a general practice."[32]

A study by Cahalan, Collette, and Hilmar of a thousand male medical

30 / Becker *et al.*, *Boys in White*, pp. 372–74.
31 / *Ibid.*, pp. 403–6.
32 / John H. Mount and D. G. Fish, "Canadian Medical Student Interest in General Practice and the Specialties," *Canadian Medical Association Journal*, vol. 94, April 2, 1966, p. 3.

students in the United States in 1956,[33] although not comparable with the Canadian study, provides data on the career interests of medical students in that country. When students were asked what field of specialization they would prefer if they were able to specialize, 30 per cent preferred internal medicine, 22 per cent preferred surgery, 10 per cent preferred obstetrics and gynaecology, and 10 per cent preferred paediatrics. All other individual specialties were preferred by less than 10 per cent of the students. A significant difference appeared in the orientations of students who planned to enter general practice and those who planned to specialize. The first group "were more concerned than others about doctor-patient relationships." The second group was "oriented relatively more toward the intellectual aspects of medicine, i.e., science or research or teaching, meeting challenging diagnostic problems, and also towards achieving prestige within the profession." This study also shows that "seven out of eight medical students preferred a non-salaried type of practice." Furthermore, "among the nine out of ten medical students who preferred some type of private (fee-for-service) practice, the rejection of salaried practice in any form appeared to be based primarily on a fear of restrictions and the limitations that might be imposed upon the way in which a salaried physician would practice medicine."

THE INTERN AND THE RESIDENT

The decision to specialize or enter general practice may not be resolved until the student has left medical school and entered a period of internship, the purpose of which is to provide him with clinical experience in order to prepare him for practice. His career decision during internship will determine if he goes on to further training as a resident and thereby gains specialty status. Internship consists of one year of education and training, after the completion of the four-year medical school programme, under the supervision of skilled physicians in hospitals.

Various types of internship exist: specialized, rotating, or mixed. The specialized internship provides training in one specialty, but it is usually the first of a number of subsequent years of resident training for a particular specialty. The rotating internship provides training in a number of specialized areas of medical service; the intern may spend from a few weeks to a few months on any particular service depending upon the number of services covered. The range of specialties is too wide for him to

---

33 / D. Cahalan *et al.*, "Career Interests and Expectations of U.S. Medical Students," *Journal of Medical Education*, vol. 32, no. 8, August 1957, pp. 557–63.

cover any one in depth. He must concentrate on those areas which will be of most use to him in general practice for which this type of internship prepares him. In the mixed internship, the intern spends more time on fewer services than in the rotating internship, and he may elect to spend the greater part of his training period working in one service. This arrangement allows the student more time to decide whether he should enter general or specialty practice.

During internship, whether rotating, specialized, or mixed, the student faces a further difficulty. The service demands of the hospital in which he is interning may be inconsistent with demands of his training programme. The hospital's primary responsibility is to treat the sick, and the number and type of patients requiring treatment may place heavy and sometimes excessive demands on its services. In order to meet these demands the hospital requires the services of the intern, which may interfere with his training programme. At times he may be given responsibilities for which he has not yet received sufficient educational preparation.

In his choice of a hospital in which to serve his internship the student may take a number of factors into account, but since there is competition among students for what they conceive to be the best hospitals in which to intern, the extent to which these factors are reflected in the hospital in which they actually intern depends on their success in this competition. Some of the factors which the student considers in judging the value of internship in a particular hospital are: the degree to which he will be allowed to exercise medical responsibility for patients and the amount of clinical experience he will gain, the quality and amount of teaching provided, the remuneration he will receive, the patient load of the hospital and its facilities, and the opportunity for contacts with the physicians who may help to further his career.[34] The extent to which teaching hospitals meet the student's conditions can vary widely.

If he interns in the United States the student will find that the value of internship may be weakened by conditions prevailing in the hospital.

Unlike a school of medicine in which the faculty take corporate responsibility for the educational programme, a hospital is more likely to consist of a federation of separate services in which each is responsible for its own standards and policies, with relatively little help, counsel, or criticism from other services.

An inevitable result of such highly individualistic and fragmented responsibility is that internship programmes vary widely in the extent to which they duplicate the experience already gained in the clinical clerkship, in the amount

34 / Becker *et al.*, *Boys in White*, pp. 387–91.

of routine and sometimes menial service required, and in their educational quality.[35]

Upon completion of the internship the student may be licensed to practise as a qualified physician unless he has decided to specialize in which case he enters a further period of training as a resident. The resident is a qualified physician who undertakes full-time training in one of the medical specialties for a period of at least three years in hospitals, clinics, dispensaries, and laboratories approved for that purpose by the Royal College of Physicians and Surgeons of Canada although the College does not directly control the organization and supervision of residency training. These responsibilities are left to the approved hospitals and other institutions.

The Royal College has approved two standards or levels of training and examinations for a specialty; one applies to fellowship in the College, and the other to certification by the College. The examinations for certification in a specialty are less demanding than those for fellowship.

Since the resident is expected to cover only one specialty he does not face the pressure which the intern must meet in trying to cover a number of specialty areas. On the other hand, like the intern, he may face excessive demands for his services which interfere with his educational development. Because of his superior status in the hospital hierarchy, compared with that of the intern, however, he may be able to delegate some of his additional responsibilities to the latter.

That residents are dissatisfied with their residency training is evident in a study undertaken by Fish. This study, based on interviews with residents training in English-speaking hospitals in Ontario and Quebec who were graduates of Canadian medical schools seeking certification or fellowship status in internal medicine, obstetrics and gynaecology, general surgery, paediatrics, and psychiatry indicates that residents feel that they are channelled "into an academic training programme to which they may not be seriously committed";[36] that the control of the hospital appointment system through which they gain specialty training is arbitrary; that there is greater emphasis on research in the fellowship training without a clear understanding of its purpose and method; that the examinations they will be required to write create sufficient anxiety to distort the purpose of residency training and make them examination-oriented; that the high failure rate in the examinations is due to restrictions on the number

35 / American Medical Association, *The Education of Physicians*, Report of the Citizens Commission on Graduate Medical Education, Chicago: 1966, p. 14.

36 / D. G. Fish, "The Resident's View of Residency Training in Canada," *Canadian Medical Association Journal*, vol. 95, October 1, 1966, p. 712.

of successful candidates imposed by the College, to the "closed shop" tactics of the College, to chance, to bias on the part of examiners, and to the examiners' attempts to locate gaps in the resident's knowledge; and that the services demanded of the resident by the training hospital are excessive.

CONTINUING EDUCATION

Having completed his internship or residency the physician enters the world of practice. As the demands of his practice increase he may find that he has little, if any, time to spare for the study necessary to keep abreast of those advances in medical knowledge and techniques affecting his practice. The knowledge and skills he has acquired may be inadequate to provide the quality of medical care which scientific developments have made possible. Unless his experience during his medical education has given him the incentive continually to inform himself of new developments affecting the quality of his service, he may ignore them. In the United States, for example, only 15 per cent of physicians participate in some form of continuing medical education.[37] At the University of Kansas Medical Center, however, participation by local physicians is as high as 65 per cent. Data are not available to show the extent of participation by physicians in programmes of continuing medical education in Canada. We can assume that such participation is probably no higher than that evident in the United States. Besides insufficient motivation on the part of the physicians, the lack of participation by Canadian practitioners may be due to the lack of organized continuing medical education programmes in this country. According to MacFarlane only three universities had any type of programme of this nature in 1964, although some efforts in this regard have been made by the College of General Practice of Canada which requires that its members undertake a specified number of hours of continuing medical education annually, and by the Canadian Medical Association, provincial, and local medical societies.[38]

Apparently the solution to the problems of continuing medical education for the practising physician has yet to be discovered. Whatever the solution may be, it must be based on at least two crucial elements. The first of these is the inculcation during the medical education process of an attitude towards continued learning which provides the impetus to such learning. The second element is the organization, under the auspices of university medical schools and medical associations, of arrangements,

37 / Lea Steeves, "The Need for Continuing Medical Education," *Canadian Medical Association Journal*, vol. 92, April 3, 1965, pp. 759–60.
38 / MacFarlane, *Medical Education in Canada*, pp. 148–52.

both financial and structural, which provide the means to this end. An additional element might be some type of control by the licensing and disciplinary body of the profession of the practising physician to make sure that he undertakes a stipulated amount of continuing education. Until such arrangements have been developed continuing education will remain one of the foremost challenges of medical education.

As student, intern, and resident the aspiring physician faces a number of pressures. The growing corpus of knowledge which generates specialization and the fragmentation of knowledge resulting in departmental isolation, the varying degrees of faculty commitment to teaching, difficulties in curriculum organization and in teaching methods, competition between clinical teachers and basic science teachers, and the tensions that arise in the relationship between the medical school and the affiliated teaching hospital all have an impact on the student. These pressures plus those he encounters as intern and student are part of the educational milieu of the medical school and the teaching hospital, and as such they will have consequences for the type of attitudes and values which he learns, and which regulate his behaviour as a student, as an intern, as a resident, and later as a practising physician.

4

THE ORGANIZATION OF
PRACTICE

ONE OF THE continuing myths of medicine is the traditional conception
of the form of medical practice. The Royal Commission on Health Services describes it in the following terms:

The physician's office resembled a parlour rather than a laboratory, with the
instruments and medications then available to medical practice assembled in
one corner of the room and the text books in another. It was the physician's
office, study, and examining room all in one. The physician – one of two or
three professional people in the community – was counsellor as much as professional advisor; his practice of medicine was more art than science. He alone
looked after all of the patient's ailments as well as those of the other members
of the household. In his role as general practitioner he practised the skills of the
surgeon, obstetrician, paediatrician, psychiatrist, and pharmacist, and he
mastered all the knowledge medical science had to offer.[1]

This stereotype is a distortion of the reality of present-day medical
practice, but it survives, curiously enough, despite developments in medicine and society. Since the era to which this stereotype refers, social
changes have created an awareness of the need for adjustments in our
social institutions and particularly in the organizational arrangements by
which they can adapt to the changing society. This awareness includes a
concern with more effective means of achieving goals through an assessment of the present means, and with the relationship of these goals to
those of society. But while government and particularly business are increasingly re-examining the relationship between means and ends, organized medicine, generally speaking, has been slow to follow suit, particularly in the organization of practice as the means of reaching the goal
of providing services to patients. The explanation for this resistance to
change can be seen by a comparison of the organization of practice and of
business and government.

1 / Royal Commission on Health Services, *Final Report*, vol. I, Ottawa: Queen's
Printer, 1964, pp. 229–30.

Modern business and government are organized on bureaucratic principles. A bureaucracy is a hierarchy of power in which those of higher rank have more power than those below them. The use of power serves to control and co-ordinate activities. "The ultimate justification of an administrative act, ... is that it is in line with the organization's rules and regulations, and that it has been approved – directly or by implication – by a superior rank."[2]

Medical practice has two significant elements which are in conflict with these organizing principles of modern bureaucracies. The intimate and confidential nature of the relationship between the physician and his patient, one in which the former has the ultimate responsibility for the life or death of the latter, requires for the doctor a high degree of independence and autonomy within his profession. "The ultimate justification for a professional act is that it is, to the best of the professional's knowledge, the right act. He might consult his colleagues before he acts, but the decision is his. If he errs, he still will be defended by his peers."[3]

The second element associated with the slow rate of change in the organization of medical practice is the strength of the tradition of freedom for doctors from control outside the profession; this independence, as will be shown in a later chapter, is part of the ideology of medicine.

Another factor related to the slow rate of innovation in the organization of practice is the nature of the market for medical services. Although his knowledge and influence are growing, the consumer of medical services does not have sufficient knowledge of the services to evaluate them fully and accurately when he receives them, or to know if, in fact, he needs them. This is not to suggest that the consumer possesses sufficient knowledge to evaluate effectively all the other goods and services he consumes, but he can obtain sufficient information about a substantial proportion of them for him to make a relatively rational and competent judgment. For medical services, on the other hand, as with other professional services, such as legal and educational, there appears to be no way in which the consumer can be sufficiently informed to enable him to make a competent judgment as to their standard of quality. Furthermore, medical services, unlike other professional services, have the power to cause bodily harm and possibly death. As noted in chapter 3, with the advancement of medical knowledge this power has grown as rapidly as the power to help. The growth of knowledge has also made a wider range of medical services available to the consumer, but this opportunity only makes it that much

2 / Amitai Etzioni, *Modern Organizations*, Englewood Cliffs, N.J.: Prentice-Hall, Inc., 1964, p. 77.
    3 / *Ibid.*

more difficult for him to make decisions about what he consumes or could consume.

These characteristics of medical services leave the physician in a powerful market position which enables him to resist innovation in the organization of practice if he so desires. But the slow pace of change in the organization of practice creates difficulties in the efficient delivery of medical services. The traditional general practitioner was able to provide a range of specific services – surgical, obstetrical, paediatric, psychiatric, pharmaceutical, and possibly others – all based on the existing corpus of medical knowledge. As this knowledge expanded the individual practitioner could no longer encompass it. Specialization emerged as the answer to the problem in learning, but this trend brought with it other problems, among them the lack of consensus within the medical profession concerning the future role of the general practitioner, a change in the nature of the doctor-patient relationship, an increased utilization of costly hospital facilities and equipment, and how to organize practice most effectively so as to provide optimal levels of medical care in terms of quantity and quality. In short, increased specialization created pressures for different patterns of delivery of medical care. "Today it is no longer possible, in terms of either knowledge or cost, for a single doctor to deliver a total medical product. Medical practice is inescapably an organizational process."[4] This being so, in what way would general practice fit into the emerging organizational patterns? To state this question is to postulate another, "What is general practice?" Peterson and his colleagues attempted to answer this question as follows:

A specialist or medical educator might limit it [general practice] to internal medicine, normal obstetrics, pediatrics, minor emotional diseases and minor surgery. This is reasonable but where does the general practitioner's competence stop in any field? He cannot treat all emotional disturbances but which ones should he attempt to manage? What are the common medical problems which he will need to master? What facilities and equipment are necessary or important? General practice is *terra incognita* in contrast with specialty practice where customary limitations define the field and the patients are selected.

An attempt to define or describe general practice involves study of it under varying circumstances. It may change from town to city, with the age of the doctor, with season of the year, with the number of partners or aides, with the size of the physician's income, and with many other factors. It would be necessary to know something about the doctor and his training, his patients and their diseases, his facilities, the extent of his work and any limitation

4 / Herman M. Somers and Anne R. Somers, *Doctors, Patients, and Health Insurance,* Washington: The Brookings Institution, 1961, p. 28.

imposed upon his practice. It is possible that organization within each practice might be important.[5]

These difficulties in defining general practice are reflected in the confusion in medical education circles concerning the education and professional role of the general practitioner, and are associated with a decline in the proportion of medical students choosing general practice as a career. Some reasons why medical students increasingly tend to prefer specialty practice have been noted in chapter 3. Judek shows that between 1943 and 1962 the percentage of general practitioners among active civilian physicians declined from 68.4 to 34.7. During the same period the percentage of specialists rose from 26.7 to 48.3.[6] The increasing preference for specialty practice is evident in both the United States and Canada. After they commence practice there is a tendency for medical graduates in the United States to change from general to specialty practice.[7] Judek reports that among Canadian-born physicians in Canada in 1962, nearly 26 per cent of all specialists and nearly 14 per cent of all consultants in private practice, and 22 per cent of specialists on hospital staff, first practised as general practitioners.[8]

The confusion over the future role of the general practitioner, his education, and the quality of the service he provides stimulated the College of General Practice of Canada to sponsor a study of general practice in Ontario and Nova Scotia. This study reveals the strains in the general practitioner's role: a rising demand for consultation by phone or at the physician's office "about myriads of details which no one, a generation or two ago, would have thought an adequate reason for consultation"[9] – the tyranny of the telephone in this regard is particularly obvious since the physician, not knowing if the call is urgent, cannot refuse it; the difficulty general practitioners face in arranging for time off from their practice and the long hours they must work; the restrictions imposed on the scope of the physician's hospital activities; the lack of prestige of the

5 / Osler L. Peterson *et al.*, "An Analytical Study of North Carolina General Practice, 1953–1954," *Journal of Medical Education*, vol. 31, no. 12, December 1956, part 2, p. 6.

6 / S. Judek, *Medical Manpower in Canada*, Royal Commission on Health Services, Ottawa: Queen's Printer, 1964, pp. 140–41. In the 1943 category of specialists I have included specialists, medical teaching, medical research, hospital service, and public health. In this category for 1962 I have included specialists, consultants, hospital staff specialists, research, teaching, and public health.

7 / Herman G. Weiskotten *et al.*, "Changes in Professional Careers of Physicians: An Analysis of a Resurvey of Physicians who were Graduated from Medical Colleges in 1935, 1940 and 1945," *Journal of Medical Education*, vol. 36, no. 11, November 1961, pp. 1565–86.

8 / Judek, *Medical Manpower*, p. 149.

9 / Kenneth F. Clute, *The General Practitioner*, Toronto: University of Toronto Press, 1963, p. 80.

general practitioner compared with that of the specialist; the lack of adequate educational preparation for general practice due partly to the type or depth of teaching material covered in medical school, partly to teaching methods and partly to the content of internship training; the difficulty in keeping abreast of advances in medicine; the problems of the division of professional and domestic responsibilities; and the problem of reconciling "the conflicting needs of the patient and of society, on the one hand, for good medical care at the least possible cost and of himself, on the other hand, for money with which to support his family."[10] The quality of care provided by general practitioners was a central concern of this study which found quality varied significantly.

Both in Ontario and in Nova Scotia, much excellent work is being done by general practitioners. Indeed, in some practices, as the very high scores achieved by some of the physicians indicate, we should be hard pressed to suggest any improvements. However, the figures and the clinical examples that we have given make clear that an appreciable percentage of the practices visited in each of the two provinces were seriously deficient in quality. We must emphasize that the deficiencies to which we refer were *not* lack of knowledge of the details of recently discovered drugs or lack of familiarity with the abstruse complexities of rare diseases. The deficiencies were in the fundamentals of clinical medicine – failure to take an adequate history, i.e. failure to gather, and to make use of, the information that the patient himself could provide about his disorder; failure to perform an adequate physical examination, and, in some cases, inability to distinguish between normal and abnormal physical findings; failure in the investigation and the treatment of cases, to think in terms of basic principles of biochemistry, physiology, pathology, microbiology, and pharmacology. The former group of physicians, those whom we found doing satisfactory work, may well be the pride of the medical profession; the latter group, the deficient group, is perhaps the more important, inasmuch as it is the challenge to the profession.[11]

These strains on the general practitioner have resulted in proposals by educators, practitioners, and professional associations for a re-definition of his role which will make it a more closely integrated unit in the organization of professional medical services. The proposals take four forms,

1 upgrading the GP; 2 replacing the GP by a better trained type of family or personal physician – the internist and paediatrician are the most frequently mentioned; 3 training all doctors in the philosophy and techniques of "comprehensive care"; 4 promoting an institutional environment which will facilitate a coordinated approach. These four methods are by no means mutually exclusive.[12]

10 / *Ibid.*, p. 473.
11 / *Ibid.*, p. 315.
12 / Somers and Somers, *Doctors, Patients, and Health Insurance*, pp. 33–34.

The acceptance by the profession of any one, or a combination of these proposals, requires changes in the educational preparation of the general practitioner, and possibly some change in the organization of practice.

In some Canadian medical schools students are exposed to the problems of general practice in various contexts such as the physician's office, the patient's home, public health clinics, and out-patient clinics. The new medical school at McMaster University, for example, includes a Department of Family Medicine which will provide a three-year graduate programme in family practice. Another significant development is the emphasis placed on the continuing education of the general practitioner by the College of General Practice of Canada which requires that all physicians wishing to maintain active membership in the College undertake "one hundred (100) hours of organized and approved post-graduate study in each two-year period."[13] Clute suggests that the organization of general practice be structured in such a way that the young physician entering practice does not assume responsibilities beyond his competence. This restructuring would take the form of group practice in which the young physician would demonstrate his competence to his senior colleagues, more particularly to specialists in internal medicine.[14]

Wolfe and his colleagues have questioned even more seriously the need for general practitioners in their present role.

Is the general practitioner in his present role an anachronism? Is it any longer possible for a doctor to care for a family when the family itself has become a smaller and much more mobile unit? Can an expert in community medical care be produced, even with longer periods of training, given the status and prestige hierarchies that exist within the medical profession, the compartmentalized structure of the medical school and modern hospital, and the changing expectations of patients?

Is the present general practitioner a superficial doctor, seeing many patients on a very cursory basis? Could the use of nurses, nursing assistants, physiotherapists, midwives and social workers and social worker aides shift much of the work load presently carried by doctors to persons who require much shorter periods of training?[15]

The fragmentation of medical knowledge, increasing specialization, and the resulting fragmentation of patient care, require more than a redefinition of the role of the general practitioner and his professional preparation. New organizational settings for practice are required if modern

13 / College of General Practice of Canada, *Brief Submitted to Royal Commission on Health Services*, Toronto: May 1962, p. 7.

14 / Clute, *The General Practitioner*, pp. 495–515.

15 / Samuel Wolfe *et al.*, "The Work of a Group of Doctors in Saskatchewan," *Milbank Memorial Fund Quarterly*, vol. 46, no. 1, January 1968, pp. 119–21.

medicine is to provide the benefits of which it is capable for all Canadians. But whatever organizational settings may be developed to meet this goal more effectively, they will probably impose certain strains upon the physician, some of which are evident today in the existing types of practice.

The practice of medicine today follows a variety of organizational patterns, but these may be combined into four major types: self-employed solo practice, partnership practice, group practice, and bureaucratic practice. The first three of these patterns are variations of private practice. The division between the two extremes of private and bureaucratic practice can be made on the basis of the degree of professional independence and autonomy. In the former type, these are the crucial conditions affecting the organization of practice; in the latter they are secondary to the functional requirements of the bureaucratic organization. This distinction is difficult to make because there are bureaucratic elements in every type of practice. The most formal bureaucratic type would include some, if not most, types of group practice, but, excluding group practice, the bureaucratic pattern would include physicians employed by all levels of government, universities, hospitals, and other health care bureaucracies.

According to Judek, in 1962 nearly 71 per cent of the civilian physicians in Canada (excluding those in the armed forces) followed some form of private practice.[16] However, as he points out with respect to civilian physicians, "postgraduates, fellows, senior interns, and residents formed the largest proportion (33.9 per cent) of those not in private practice."[17] Many of these would subsequently enter private practice thus increasing the percentage in this type of practice.

Table 6 indicates the extent to which physicians tend to transfer from one type of practice to another during their professional careers. Of all physicians who had first entered private practice, 91 per cent remained in 1962. However, of all physicians who had first entered what we have termed bureaucratic practice only 74.2 per cent remained in 1962; over 25 per cent had switched to private practice. In other words, in 1962 there appeared to have been more movement from bureaucratic to private practice than in the opposite direction. This tendency is also evident in the United States.[18] There is a difference between Canadian-born and immigrant physicians in this regard. Of all immigrant physicians who

16 / Judek, *Medical Manpower*, p. 144.
17 / *Ibid.*, p. 147.
18 / Weiskotten *et al.*, "Professional Careers of Physicians," p. 1584.

TABLE 6
Percentage Distribution for Canada of Active Canadian-Born and Immigrant Physicians by Type of First Practice and Type of Practice in which Engaged in 1962 (N = 9,968)

	Type of present (1962) practice		
Type of first practice	Private	Bureaucratic and other	Total
Private	91.0	9.0	100
Canadian-born	92.2	7.8	100
Immigrant	86.7	13.3	100
Bureaucratic and other	25.8	74.2	100
Canadian-born	23.2	76.8	100
Immigrant	30.3	69.7	100
Total	78.2	21.8	100

SOURCE: S. Judek, *Medical Manpower in Canada*, Royal Commission on Health Services, Ottawa: Queen's Printer, 1964, pp. 149–50.

first entered private practice 86.7 per cent remained in 1962 compared with 92.2 per cent of Canadian-born physicians. On the other hand, of all immigrant physicians who first entered bureaucratic practice 69.7 per cent remained in 1962 compared with 76.8 per cent of Canadian-born physicians.

Table 7 shows that of the number of civilian physicians in private practice in 1962 over 67 per cent were in solo practice, nearly 19 per cent in

TABLE 7
Percentage Distribution for Canada of Active Physicians in Private Practice by Type of Practice and Type of Work, 1962 (N = 7,751)

	Type of work		
Type of practice	General practitioner	Specialist*	Total
Solo	67.0	67.5	67.2
Partnership	20.4	17.3	18.9
Group practice	12.6	15.2	13.9
Total	100.0	100.0	100.0

*Includes consultants.
SOURCE: S. Judek, *Medical Manpower in Canada*, Royal Commission on Health Services, Ottawa: Queen's Printer, 1964, p. 145.

TABLE 8
Percentage Distribution for Canada of Physicians by Year First Licensed to Practise in Canada by Type of Practice, 1962 (N = 11,382)

Type of practice	Year first licensed to practise in Canada										
	Pre 1923	1923–27	1928–32	1933–37	1938–42	1943–47	1948–52	1953–57	1958 and later	Not given	Total
Self	86.4	80.8	76.2	71.7	70.0	67.9	66.4	62.0	54.3	78.0	67.2
Partnership	5.6	7.9	14.1	16.1	17.9	18.8	20.6	22.1	23.9	10.2	18.6
Group	7.9	11.4	9.7	12.2	12.2	13.2	13.0	15.8	21.7	11.8	14.1
Total private	99.9	100.1	100.0	100.0	100.1	99.9	100.0	99.9	99.9	100.0	99.9
Private	82.1	71.6	70.7	72.5	78.9	76.5	74.6	69.8	49.1	35.8	67.1
Bureaucratic*	17.9	28.4	29.3	27.5	21.1	23.5	25.4	30.2	50.9	64.2	32.9
Total private and bureaucratic	100.0	100.0	100.0	100.0	100.0	100.0	100.0	100.0	100.0	100.0	100.0

*"Bureaucratic" includes: hospitals; Department of National Health and Welfare; Department of Veterans Affairs; Canadian Pension Commission; regular armed forces; Defence Research Board; Department of National Defence; Department of Justice; other federal departments, boards, agencies; provincial departments of health; provincial hospital insurance administrations; provincial departments of education; workmen's compensation boards; other provincial departments, boards, agencies; counties or municipalities; universities or colleges; industry; Medical Research Council; voluntary agencies; pharmaceutical companies; life insurance companies; prepaid medical care and hospital plans.

SOURCE: Royal Commission on Health Services, Survey of Physicians in Canada, 1962.

partnership, and just under 14 per cent in group practice.[19] Obviously, solo practice is the type preferred by a majority of civilian physicians in private practice regardless of whether they are general practitioners or specialists.

Although physicians tend to remain in private practice once having entered it there is, nevertheless, an increasing tendency for younger physicians to enter bureaucratic, as opposed to private, practice. The first line of Table 8 shows a steadily decreasing proportion of physicians entering private and solo practice. Comparing the proportion of physicians in private solo practice who were first licensed prior to 1923 with the proportion in this type of practice who were first licensed in 1958 and later, there is a substantial decline from over 86 per cent to over 54 per cent. This decline is accompanied by the increasing proportion of physicians who enter other forms of private practice more closely approximating the bureaucratic type. Thus, the proportion of physicians entering a private partnership steadily increased from over 5 per cent for those first licensed prior to 1923 to nearly 24 per cent for those first licensed in 1958 and later. Similarly, those entering private group practice increased from nearly 8 per cent to around 22 per cent during the same period.

The purest bureaucratic type of practice, as noted above, is that found in government, universities, and industry. When the various private forms of practice are combined, as in the last few lines of Table 8, and compared with the bureaucratic form, the proportion entering this latter type, according to the year first licensed, increased from nearly 18 per cent for those first licensed prior to 1923 to nearly 51 per cent in 1958 and later. This latter percentage is probably inflated by numbers of interns and residents taking training in hospitals. Nevertheless, it is a fairly safe assumption that the true figure is between 30 and 51 per cent, and there can be little doubt that there is a trend towards the bureaucratic form.

TYPES OF PRACTICE AND ROLE STRAINS

Each of the three major patterns of private practice designated above as solo, partnership, and group, and the bureaucratic form of practice have a particular structure which may create strains for the physician as he seeks to perform his role. The nature and severity of these strains depend, to a large extent, on the pattern of practice. Some are more obvious, and possibly more severe, in some types of practice than in others. Some, for example, such as the kind of control exercised by colleagues, are common to all, and all are related, either directly or indirectly, to the cost, quality, and availability of care.

19 / Judek, *Medical Manpower*, p. 145.

Solo practice is the practice of medicine by a general practitioner or a specialist who assumes the responsibility for providing those services for which he has been trained, through either formal education or experience, or both, and who is recognized by his professional licensing body and his professional peers as competent to provide these services. This responsibility includes the provision of technical facilities and equipment plus the organization of an office with the nursing, paramedical, and clerical staff whom the practitioner considers necessary for the effective provision of his services. He may thus face a substantial initial financial investment in establishing his office and continuing heavy overhead costs.

The physician in solo practice must also attract a clientele and maintain an active association with a hospital to whose services he is allowed access for the diagnosis and treatment of his patients. As we have noted already, if he is a general practitioner he may be restricted by a hospital Medical Advisory Committee in the type of services he can provide for his patients in hospital.

Within limits, the solo practitioner is responsible for the cost, availability, and quality of services he provides, and in assuming this responsibility he thereby maintains his professional autonomy. On the other hand, the physician practising under this autonomous, fee-for-service arrangement faces certain pressures which can have repercussions on the cost, quality, and availability of care he provides.

In this type of practice the physician can determine his income. It is based on the amount of work he wishes to undertake and on the fees suggested by his professional association and agreed to by third parties such as insurance companies and voluntary, sometimes physician-sponsored, prepayment plans, which attempt to protect individuals from some, if not all, of the financial hazards of illness. He can charge more, or less, than the suggested fee schedule, depending on his assessment of the financial ability of the patients, but if he charges more than the fee agreed to by any third parties involved, he must bill the patient for the additional amount.

A study published by the Department of National Health and Welfare in 1967 shows that between 1957 and 1965 the average gross annual earnings of "active civilian physicians whose main employment is the provision of personal medical care services and whose professional income derives primarily from fees for services rendered"[20] rose from $20,804 to $32,799, but during the same period average annual expenses of practice increased from $7,952 to $10,735. The average expenses of practice as a percentage of average gross earning declined from 38.2 to 32.7 in

20 / Canada, Department of National Health and Welfare, *Earnings of Physicians in Canada, 1957–1965*, Ottawa: 1967, p. iii.

this period which resulted in average net earnings rising from $12,852 to $22,064.[21] This study shows an interesting change in the sources of payments of these physicians during this period. Payment from the private sector, comprising direct payments from patients and from voluntary medical care insurance plans, as a percentage of all payments, declined slightly from 88.3 to 86.8; payment from the public sector, comprising public medical care insurance plans, government payments for individuals, and workmen's compensation boards, rose from 11.7 per cent to 13.2 per cent. Of the changes in the private sector, the direct payments from patients as a percentage of total payments declined from 53.9 to 31.3 and payments from voluntary medical care plans rose from 34.4 to 55.5. Evidently, during the period 1957–65 payments to physicians by third parties for services to patients, as a percentage of all payments to physicians, increased from 46.1 to 68.7.[22]

Since the private physician's income is dependent upon the fees he charges for particular services and the number of patients he treats, in order to increase his income he must either raise his fees or increase the number of patients he serves. If the former action does not result in the desired financial return, he must rely on the latter, but this may mean that he is so pressured by the demands of the increased load of patients he may not be readily available for all cases demanding his services, or he may attempt to see all who seek his services but deal with them more quickly than he would with fewer patients; he thereby creates less satisfaction for the patient and for himself as well as lowering the quality of care. Data collected by the Royal Commission on Health Services in 1962 indicate that the average weekly patient load of 88 for general practitioners in solo practice was higher than that for general practitioners in either partnership or group practice with 84 and 77 respectively.[23] Despite this larger average weekly patient load, the average annual total net income of these general practitioners which in 1960 stood at $13,820 was appreciably below that of their medical colleagues in group practice, who, with fewer patients, earned an average net income of $19,420.[24] But the application of modern medical knowledge to patient care in many cases requires more time per patient than ever before. The financial pressure to see as many patients as possible, therefore, may contribute to a lowering of the standard of care. The structure of the fee schedule may also contribute to this result. In their 1964 study of the Saskatoon Community Health Services

21 / *Ibid.*, p. 1.
22 / *Ibid.*, p. 14.
23 / Royal Commission on Health Services, Survey of Physicians in Canada, 1962.
24 / Judek, *Medical Manpower*, p. 221.

Medical Clinic, a consumer-sponsored organization in which physicians are remunerated on a fee-for-service basis by the Saskatchewan Medical Care Insurance Commission, Wolfe and his colleagues found that the fee-for-service schedule paid the general practitioner in the clinic "too well for doing procedures that other doctors can do better, and pays him very poorly indeed for just those services at which he should excel."[25]

Financial pressure may also hinder, if not prevent, the physician from acquiring new medical knowledge, either through continuous informal study, or more formally through continuing education programmes organized by medical schools, medical societies, or other bodies. Understandably, this difficulty in keeping abreast of medical knowledge could lower the quality of medical care.

Since, in the present state of medical knowledge, no physician can know all there is to know about many of his patients' illnesses, he should refer problem cases to his professional colleagues who are more competent than he in certain areas. Friedson points out pressures that stem from this arrangement which may interfere with adequate consultation:

A truly autonomous fee-for-service arrangement is inherently unstable, however: it is eventually bound to fall under the control of either patients or colleagues. In a system of free competition the physician may neither count on the loyalty of his patients (with whom he has no contract) nor on that of his colleagues (with whom he has no ties and who are competing with him). Since his colleagues are competitors, he is not likely to solicit their advice or trade information and he certainly will not refer his patients to them for consultations. Under these circumstances, he is quite isolated from his colleagues and relatively free of their control – but at the same time he is very vulnerable to control by his clients. To keep them, he must give them what they want, or someone else will attract them away by doing so. Obviously, conscientious practice under these conditions is difficult and frustrating.[26]

The lack of observation of the solo practitioner's professional conduct by his peers means that there is a minimum of professional control over the quality of the services he provides, particularly outside the hospital. On the other hand, referrals and consultations, although increasing the degree of observability of his professional activities by his peers and thereby creating pressure upon him to maintain high standards of medical care, make available to his patients a wider range of services than he alone can provide and thus increase their medical care costs. Furthermore, since the referral of patients to a range of specialists will tend to decrease

25 / Wolfe *et al.*, "A Group of Doctors in Saskatchewan," p. 118.
26 / Eliot Freidson, "The Organization of Medical Practice," in H. E. Freeman *et al.* (eds.), *Handbook of Medical Sociology*, Englewood Cliffs, N.J.: Prentice-Hall, Inc., 1963, p. 303.

the patient's "attachment" to the solo practitioner, it thereby places a strain on the doctor-patient relationship. In addition, such referrals will fragment the care of the patient with consequent loss of the "over-all view" by the practitioner.

In solo practice these pressures affecting the cost, quality, and availability of medical care, and particularly what Friedson terms" client control"[27] of the doctor have resulted in co-operative forms of practice. These, which are more than simple referral arrangements, have lessened professional autonomy by increasing "colleague control"[28] of the individual doctor.

Co-operative practice may consist of a series of informal arrangements between a number of physicians or it may be a more formal organizational pattern such as is evident in group practice (discussed below). Hall describes the informal co-operative system as consisting of a colleague network which controls both the allocation of hospital privileges in those hospitals in which the members hold dominant positions and patient referrals.[29] Lacking membership in such an informal colleague network, the solo practitioner competing with one would be hard-pressed to operate his practice effectively, but, on the other hand, as a member of such a group he places himself under a degree of colleague control. Such a membership is nevertheless almost a necessary element of practice, and the idea of a completely independent solo medical practitioner is thus more of a myth than a reality.

One form of co-operative practice is the partnership based on "a legal agreement between two or more physicians which provides for mutual responsibility to their patients and to each other."[30] The legal rights and obligations are sustained by common law. Such a partnership consists of two or more physicians and stipulates specific rights, duties, and obligations for its members. Major decisions affecting the partnership group may be made by all group members, but the medical and other privileges of junior partners may be restricted until full partnership is achieved. Some partnerships may be departmentalized in that the partnership group is divided into separate units each representing a separate area of medicine. Each department consists of two or more physicians who share the facilities necessary to practise their specialty. The concentration of professional authority within the department lessens the possibility of a centrali-

27 / *Ibid.*

28 / *Ibid.*

29 / Oswald Hall, "The Informal Organization of the Medical Profession," *Canadian Journal of Economics and Political Science*, vol. 12, February 1946, pp. 30–44.

30 / As quoted in E. P. Jordan (ed.), *The Physician and Group Practice*, Chicago: Year Book Publishers Inc., 1958, p. 20.

zation of administrative authority in such a group. Like other forms of co-operative practice, such as association or group practice, the partnership usually provides for extended leaves for study or other types of leave which help the practitioner to maintain, and sometimes improve, his level of competence.

An association is more formally organized than a partnership. Policies and administrative procedures are usually laid down by an elected board of governors. These cover matters such as the nature of the organization, the identity of association members, and recruitment. Each member is given specific responsibilities which are indicated in a contractual agreement between the association and the member. This agreement also covers matters dealing with the separation of members whether this be by resignation, retirement, or discharge.

As noted previously, group practice is the most bureaucratized form of private practice. According to Jordan, "Group Medical Practice is the application of medical service by a number of physicians working in systematic association with the joint use of equipment and technical personnel and with centralized administration and financial organization."[31] Although each of the forms of practice already discussed contains bureaucratic elements, these are more prevalent in the various patterns of group practice, and of course, still more so in the completely bureaucratized practice evident, for example, in government-controlled medical and other health services.

In group practice, as in the pure bureaucratic pattern, there is a division between professional and administrative power and responsibility and conflicts may occur when decisions need to be made concerning the relative importance of professional and administrative responsibilities. But whereas in group practice professional considerations are likely to predominate in decisions regarding the provision and administration of medical services, within the pure bureaucratic type of practice such decisions will probably be based on administrative considerations.

Medical personnel in group practice may be under the professional authority of a medical director, with the administrative and non-technical personnel under the authority of a business administrator. In some groups a physician may have superior authority in both professional and administrative fields. In a large group practice a governing body may be set up in both of these fields, the decisions of each being implemented by an executive committee.

31 / *Ibid.*, p. 20. For a discussion of the difficulties involved in an attempt to define group practice see, J. A. Boan, *Group Practice*, Royal Commission on Health Services, Ottawa: Queen's Printer, 1966, pp. 71–73.

Group practice may be classified according to the type of service offered ranging from the services provided by general practitioners only to those provided by specialists only with the same or different areas of competence. Groups may also provide comprehensive medical care through the spectrum of services offered by both general practitioners and specialists sharing facilities and diagnostic equipment. Some groups provide care to individuals for only one, or a number of, episodes of illness. One well-known example of such a group is the Mayo Clinic. Other types of groups classified by Jordan are "diagnostic groups," which provide only examination and consultation services, and "institutional groups," which are organized within a medical school or a hospital to assist in the teaching and in the practice of medicine.[32]

Of particular interest in Canada are the community health clinics which were organized in some communities in the Province of Saskatchewan during, and subsequent to, the dispute between the government and the physicians of that province in 1962. These clinics are incorporated under the Saskatchewan Mutual and Hospital Benefit Association Act with the aim of providing medical services in a co-operative manner. The community "provides the premises on a rental basis."[33] Each clinic has a board of governors elected annually consisting of representatives of the public served by the clinic and its physicians. Comprehensive coverage of medical services is achieved through referrals between physicians within the clinic. If particular services are not available within the clinic outside referrals are made. Patients using these services may change from one physician to another in the clinic if they are not satisfied. A significant element in this form of group practice organization is that the clientele is given a role to play in the formulation of policies governing its administration and in the planning of the services it provides.

Another interesting development in group practice in Canada was inaugurated by the Sault Ste Marie Group Health Association sponsored by the local of the United Steelworkers of America. The Association organized a group of union members at the Algoma Steel Plant plus members of other unions. It hired a medical director who was given the responsibility for hiring physicians to staff the Center as salaried employees of the Association. As the organization developed the original group of premium-paying union members was expanded to include private fee-paying patients. This expansion, plus the introduction of the Ontario Medical Services Insurance Plan paying for physicians' services on a fee-for-service basis, brought about a change in organization which made it

32 / Jordan, *The Physician and Group Practice*, pp. 26–32.
33 / Boan, *Group Practice*, p. 12.

possible for all individuals, regardless of whether they were insured or not insured, to use the services of the Center. In 1966 the physicians employed by the Association formed a partnership. They use the Center and receive a percentage of the premiums paid to the Association besides retaining all fee-for-service income.

Some proponents of group practice have claimed that it lowers the cost, raises the quality, and increases the availability of medical services. Available evidence suggests that when compared with solo practice the range of facilities and services usually found in group practice enables the physician to treat a greater proportion of his patients on an ambulatory basis rather than in hospital thus saving costly hospital bed days. As Boan points out, however, "the claim that group medical practice reduces hospital costs relies on the fact that a certain percentage of patients can be treated on an ambulatory basis. Obviously this does not eliminate all costs. It shifts some of them from the community to the patient or his family."[34] There is some evidence to suggest that group practice improves the quality of care. As we have pointed out, the observability of his professional activities by his peers provides the physician with an incentive to meet their standards. Knowing their expectations of his performance, and wishing to meet with their approval and approbation, the physician tries to meet these expectations. Furthermore, group practice provides opportunities for easy consultation and allocation of responsibilities, which in turn allows the physician time for continuing education; both of these advantages can contribute to maintaining the quality of medical care. Boan claims that the productivity of physicians in group practice is higher than that of those in solo practice.

This means that medical services of comparable quality can be provided at a lower real cost in a group setting than they can under conditions of solo practice. These gains can be attributed to the fact that the practice is organized to take advantage of specialization and division of labour, to use capital equipment efficiently, and to avoid the costly misuse of time that many solo practitioners fall heir to.[35]

Apparently, then, group practice tends to lower the costs due to hospitalization by decreasing the rate of hospital admissions and possibly the length of hospital stay. One would also expect it to maintain standards by increasing the observability of the physician's activities by his peers, and it probably increases the availability of medical care by increasing the physician's productivity. However, the data available at present indicate only that group practice lowers the hospitalization rate of group

34 / *Ibid.*, p. 2.
35 / *Ibid.*, p. 5.

practice patients. Objective and systematic comparative studies of the benefits in terms of cost, quality, and availability of medical care provided by group and other forms of practice are required before the advantages, and disadvantages, of various forms of practice can be determined. That such studies have not been undertaken may seem surprising in view of the emphasis on scientific experiment in modern medicine, which would lead some observers to expect the profession to be willing to experiment to a much greater extent than is now evident with various forms of practice not only to determine their merits in terms of the above factors but also to ascertain their effect on professional autonomy. However, there are at least two major obstacles to this type of experimentation and innovation. Until recently the vocational pattern existing in Canadian medical schools in which large numbers of private practitioners served as part-time teachers acted as a brake on experiments in ways of organizing practice: their influence has tended to perpetuate the pattern of their own practice. Furthermore, the strong adherence to the fee-for-service system of remuneration provides an effective obstacle to any new ways of organizing practice that may include new forms of remuneration.

There can be little doubt that professional autonomy is more restricted in group practice than in solo practice for in the former the integration of a physician's services with those of his colleagues who are members of the same group practice makes that physician open to a higher degree of control by his colleagues than a solo practice physician experiences. As we shall show in the following chapter, all physicians practising in a hospital are more or less under observation by their colleagues practising there, notably through the hospital medical advisory committee and its subcommittees such as the tissue committee, but in the part of his practice carried on outside the hospital the solo practitioner can insulate himself from colleague observation and control to a greater extent than the physician in group practice. What degree of professional autonomy is compatible with a set of practice arrangements that will ensure optimum cost, quality, and availability? This is a question that all client-oriented professions must face as technical advances make present practice arrangements increasingly difficult to rationalize in social or economic terms.

The pure form of bureaucratic practice is found in government and in those community agencies in which the physician is under the control of an administrative or non-professional authority in a system of hierarchical co-ordination designed to achieve the aims of the organization. Modern industrial societies require bureaucratic organizations and professional specialization, and both bureaucracies and professions require sets of rules or codes which govern the behaviour of their members. Within the bureaucratic organization there is a division of labour in which the rights, duties, and responsibilities of particular offices are specified in a set of rules. In order to attain its goals the bureaucracy requires a high degree of centralized planning with orders coming down from the top. The superior authority of those in high offices legitimizes the orders they issue to those below them in the hierarchy of offices. Behaviour is based on the rules of office and the orders issued by those in positions of superior authority. As Porter points out: "Success depends on carrying out orders, so that bureaucratically organized workers are predisposed to obedience. The bureaucratic structure of offices also represents the career avenues for those who want to rise. Obedience and the observance of rules improve the chances of promotion. Sanctions and rewards, like orders, also come from the top down."[36]

The physician, however, like other professionals, governs his actions according to his determination of the interests of his patients: his authority is based on his technical competence and his central concern as a professional is service to patients. The authority of the bureaucrat is a function of the office he holds and his actions are directed to furthering the goals of the organization. The physician working in a pure type of bureaucracy or in a bureaucratized type of practice therefore is controlled to a large extent by those in supervisory offices above him and by the rules of the organization. Thus, he faces conflicting pressures resulting from the incompatibility of his professional and bureaucratic roles.

The tension which this incompatibility can create may be evident, for example, in a physician's relations with his patients. Solomon explains this situation succinctly:

The independent professional determines the fee to be charged for his services, serves many clients, and can always afford to lose a few. The employed professional may serve numerous clients, but even if he does, his employer sets the fee for services, and the professional receives a salary which is determined by the operation of the labour market in which he offers himself. This is by no means the whole story, but it suggests a crucial aspect. The employer is a powerful intermediary between the professional and his clients, and the professional may frequently have to choose between the interests of employer and client.[37]

36 / John Porter, *The Vertical Mosaic*, Toronto: University of Toronto Press, 1965, p. 220.

37 / David N. Solomon, "Professional Persons in Bureaucratic Organizations," *Symposium on Preventive and Social Psychiatry*, sponsored jointly by the Walter Reed Army Institute of Research, the Walter Reed Army Medical Center, and the National Research Council, Washington: us Government Printing Office, 1958, pp. 255–56.

As Solomon suggests, one of the crucial elements in the organization of practice is the degree of control by the physician over the system of remuneration. The extent of this type of control illustrates one of the major difficulties facing the medical profession, which seeks to maintain a maximum degree of professional autonomy for the practising physician in an era when the main source of funds for the payment of his services is likely to be the public treasury. The physician realizes that such a source is open to public scrutiny, accountability, and control since "he who pays the piper calls the tune"; he is therefore anxious to determine the form that such control will take for it could severely restrict, if not destroy, his professional autonomy as he at present conceives it.

Different systems of remuneration provide opportunities for more or less interference in the relationship between physicians and patients. Salaried positions are an integral element in a bureaucratic structure in which the employer has the power to interfere in this relationship; the fee-for-service is associated with independent practice in which there is less opportunity for outside interference. This is not to suggest, however, that a combination of these two methods of remuneration, and others, is not feasible in these contexts. The prevailing systems of remuneration in different countries show the extent to which combinations of different systems in different types of practice are possible.

Abel-Smith discusses the development of different systems of remuneration in different countries in terms of the power of the consumer relative to the power of the provider of medical care. In his words,

Much has depended on who produced first a strong organization – the patient or the doctor? Much has depended also on political lobbying power. The actual systems adopted have varied not only because of differences in the strength of "opposing" interests but also because of diverse interpretations of where self-interest lay, the type of doctor holding power in the professional group, and such factors as levels of living and population density.[38]

The various methods of remunerating the physician range from salary, through *capitation* (see below), to fee-for-service; the last-named method can be divided into fee-for-service systems in which there is a direct financial relationship between physician and patients, with, in some cases, the patient subsequently being reimbursed, in whole or in part, by a third party, and fee-for-service systems in which the physician is paid directly by a third party.[39]

38 / Brian Abel-Smith, "Paying the Family Doctor," *Medical Care*, vol. 1, no. 1, January–March 1963, p. 28.
39 / J. Hogarth, "Paying the General Practitioner: The Comparison with Europe," *Medical Care*, vol. 1, no. 1, January–March 1963, p. 23.

In the salaried method of payment, the physician is paid by the organization of which he is a member and which specifies the conditions of employment and the amount to be paid. Under this system the degree of strain felt by the physician depends to a large extent on the strength with which he holds the tradition of professional autonomy and independance with its associated attitudes, and its possible conflict with the organizational demands of modern scientific medicine of which one element is the salaried method of payment.

In the capitation system of payment the physician is given a set fee for providing his services to a patient for a specified length of time. This system is generally used only for the remuneration of general practitioners, with specialists coming under some other system of remuneration. According to Roemer, "the real *modus operandi* of capitation payment ... assumes general practitioners working more or less independently in separate offices."[40] In other words, since this method of payment is not imbedded in a bureaucratic context, it assures the physician of a guaranteed income with a minimum of bureaucratic interference with his professional autonomy. Although evidence is lacking, Glaser believes that neglect of the patient does not occur in those countries using this system. As he says,

Certain important countervailing forces protect the patient, such as the individual doctor's ethical conscience, the medical profession's group opinion condemning dereliction of duty, and the danger of official complaints and lawsuits. But possibly capitation may result in transfers to services outside the G.P.'s panel practice. For example, the G.P. may refer the time-consuming patient to another organization ... unless administrative controls exist.[41]

The fee-for-service system of physician remuneration is the payment to a physician by the patient, or by a third party on his behalf, for the servies rendered by the physician. Under this arrangement the physician determines the fee as well as the services for which it is paid. It is, of course, true that the decision regarding the fee to be charged is not based solely on the basis of his assessment of the price to be charged for the services he provides. His assessment may be affected by a published fee schedule, by custom, or by supply and demand, but whatever the factors affecting his decision may be, the final determination of price is his responsibility.[42] In Canada and the United States this method of paying for

40 / Milton I. Roemer, "On Paying the Doctor and the Implications of Different Methods," *Journal of Health and Human Behaviour*, vol. 3, no. 1, Spring 1962, p. 10.
41 / William A. Glaser, *The Compensation of Physicians*, Columbia University, Bureau of Applied Social Research, September 1963, mimeo., pp. 11–85.
42 / Roemer, "On Paying the Doctor," p. 6.

physicians' services is traditionally associated with private independent practice and professional autonomy. It is also associated with the "free enterprise system" by its most vociferous proponents who proclaim the advantages of "free enterprise medicine" over all other systems of providing medical care.

TABLE 9
Percentage Distribution for Canada of Physicians by Type of Remuneration by Type of Practice, 1962 (N = 10,993)

Type of practice	Type of remuneration			
	Fees	Salary	Other	Total
Self	97.5	0.5	2.0	100.0
Partnership	95.2	4.3	0.4	99.9
Group	80.6	18.9	0.5	100.0
Bureaucracy*	6.7	87.7	5.7	100.1
(Other, not given)	9.3	79.6	11.1	100.0

*"Bureaucracy" includes: hospitals; Department of National Health and Welfare; Department of Veterans Affairs; Canadian Pension Commision; regular armed forces; Defence Research Board; Department of National Defence; Department of Justice; other federal departments, boards, agencies; provincial department of health; provincial hospital insurance administrations; provincial department of education; workmen's compensation board; other provincial departments, boards, agencies; counties or municipalities; universities or colleges; industry; Medical Research Council; voluntary agencies; pharmaceutical companies; life insurance companies; prepaid medical care and hospital plans.

SOURCE: Royal Commission on Health Services, Survey of Physicians in Canada, 1962.

It is obvious from Table 9 that in private practice – self, partnership, or group – the overwhelming majority of physicians in 1962 were remunerated through a fee-for-service arrangement. Of the physicians in solo (self) practice over 97 per cent were paid by the fee-for-service arrangement. In partnership practice over 95 per cent, and in group practice over 80 per cent, were remunerated in this manner.

There is evidence, however, which suggests that the salary method of remuneration is less objectionable to younger than to older physicians. Table 10 shows that an increasing proportion of young physicians are practising under the salary method of payment. These data can be related to those in Table 8 which indicate that an increasing proportion of younger physicians prefer a bureaucratic form of practice. Table 10 indicates that in 1964, of those physicians first licensed to practice in the period 1948–52 or subsequently, an increasing proportion preferred the salary method, or at least were not averse to working in a bureaucracy where they were

TABLE 10
Percentage Distribution of Physicians by Type of Remuneration and Year
First Licensed to Practise in Canada, 1961 (N = 10,993)

Year first licensed to practise in Canada	Type of remuneration			
	Fees	Salary	Other	Total
Pre 1923	75.4	19.0	5.6	100.0
1923–27	69.8	27.5	2.7	100.0
1928–32	69.7	27.8	2.5	100.0
1933–37	71.6	25.9	2.5	100.0
1938–42	80.5	17.5	2.0	100.0
1943–47	78.0	19.8	2.2	100.0
1948–52	74.7	22.9	2.4	100.0
1953–57	69.0	28.1	2.9	100.0
1958 and later	42.6	53.9	3.5	100.0
Not given	37.5	57.9	4.6	100.0
Total	65.9	31.1	2.9	99.9

SOURCE: Royal Commission on Health Services, Survey of Physicians
in Canada, 1962.

paid by salary. The proportion working under this method of payment
rose from nearly 23 per cent between 1948 and 1952 to nearly 54 per
cent between 1958 and 1962. This latter figure may be inflated by a
number of young physicians who were licensed but who were undertaking
further studies, and probably were remunerated by some form of salary
arrangement.

The four major patterns of service noted above – self-employed solo
practice, partnership practice, group practice, and bureaucratic practice –
all have functional consequences for their participating physicians. Some
of the particular consequences of the different patterns have been described above, but some of these are common to all patterns. The severity
of these consequences for the physician, however, seems to increase according to the extent to which a pattern of practice is bureaucratized.
Nevertheless, although a significant proportion of the profession prefer to
practise according to their conception of a traditional solo practice, a
growing proportion are willing to practise under varying degrees of
co-operative practice including its most highly bureaucratized form. This
suggests that group practice may be seen by some physicians as a means
whereby they can retain a high degree of professional independence and
autonomy while at the same time maximizing the opportunities to practise
modern scientific medicine of high quality which requires a degree of
bureaucratic organization.

Judek provides evidence for this statement. He shows that over 81 per cent of physicians in partnership practice and 91 per cent in group practice think that group practice improves the quality of medical services. Of those in solo practice over 46 per cent are of the same opinion; nearly 50 per cent, however, of this group do not think that group practice has this result. Evidently, despite the fact that they are actually engaged in solo practice, close to 50 per cent of solo practitioners realize their mode of practice could be improved with a greater degree of bureaucratization. No matter how long they had been in practice, over 60 per cent of all physicians in this survey claimed that group practice improves the quality of medical services. The majority of these physicians also claimed that group practice improves the availability of medical services, the proportions ranging from just over 70 per cent of those in solo practice to over 95 per cent of those in group practice. Regardless of the duration of practice most felt the same way although there was an increasingly higher proportion with this opinion as the duration of practice decreased, the range being from a high of nearly 83 per cent of those who had been in practice less than ten years to just over 71 per cent of those who had been in practice forty years or more. When these physicians were asked if group practice improved the working conditions of physicians even higher proportions answered in the affirmative, the range here being from over 87 per cent of those in solo practice to just over 98 per cent in group practice, and from nearly 94 per cent of those whose duration of practice was less than ten years to 84 per cent whose length of practice was forty years and over.[43] These data would seem to indicate that regardless of the manner in which they now practice and the length of time they have been in practice the majority of physicians recognize the gains to be derived from at least one form of bureaucratic practice in terms of improvement in availability of services and in physicians' working conditions.

Despite these, and possibly other advantages, the foregoing analysis has shown that bureaucratic practice, of which group practice is one form, imposes serious strains in the present-day physician's performance of his role, strains which are expressed, as we shall show in a later chapter, in the ideology of organized medicine.

43 / Judek, *Medical Manpower*, p. 213.

5

THE HOSPITAL

THE MODERN HOSPITAL plays a central role in medical care. Fifty or more years ago a hospital was viewed by many as a refuge or as a place to die, rather than as a treatment centre. Today it is the focus of community health care, the physician's work shop, an educational centre, and a centre for medical research.

Hospitals in Canada are operated by six types of agencies with the day-to-day responsibility for ensuring ability to provide service. These comprise voluntary bodies who may own and operate hospitals on a non-profit basis; municipalities such as a city, town, county, or other forms of municipal government which are empowered to levy taxes; provincial governments; the federal government; industry; and proprietary bodies. The last named, the so-called private hospitals which can be owned by an individual or group on a profit-making basis, are not the concern of this analysis which is focussed on the public hospitals.

Hospital care in Canada is financed under the provisions of the Hospital Insurance and Diagnostic Services legislation of 1958 whereby the federal and provincial governments share the cost of provincially administered hospital insurance programmes. These programmes are an attempt on the part of the two levels of government to meet the problems raised by increased utilization of hospitals, significant advances in the treatment of disease with the accompanying complex technology, changing attitudes towards hospital care on the part of physicians and patients, and the cost and availability of hospital resources.

In Canada between 1948 and 1964 the estimated number of acute treatment hospital beds set up rose from 60,077 to 101,953, or from 4.6 to 5.3 per thousand population.[1] During the same period the estimated number of chronic and convalescent hospital beds set up rose from 6,714 to 19,317, or from 0.5 to 1.0 per thousand population. As noted earlier (p. 12), this seventeen-year period saw hospital admissions rise from

1 / Canada, Department of National Health and Welfare, *The Economies and Costs of Health Care*, Ottawa: 1967, p. 17.

111 to 152 per thousand population and the average length of stay per case increase from 10.0 to 10.2 days for general hospitals, and decrease from 311.5 to 224.6 days for chronic hospitals and from 56.3 to 40.5 days for convalescent hospitals. At the same time, the days of care per thousand population rose substantially from 1,318 to 1,759 and the operating expenditures per patient day of care from $7.88 to $29.18.[2]

HOSPITAL ORGANIZATION

The modern hospital is a much more complex social organization than most of our present-day enterprises; "... partly by rational design, partly by the inheritance of historical accident, the hospital entails a multiplicity of goals, a riotous profusion of personnel, and an extremely fine-grained division of labour."[3] The relationship between this complexity and the role strain of the physician can be understood if the institution is viewed as sets or "clusters of role relationships, of those recurring nexuses of interpersonal action which center around some desired end."[4] The central purpose of the diverse activities carried on in the hospital is the treatment of the patient on whom are focussed, directly or indirectly, the activities of hospital personnel.

The modern hospital has a governing body which is responsible for the policies of the institution in relation to the health needs of the community, for providing the necessary facilities and equipment, for maintaining adequate levels of patient care by professional staff, and for adequate hospital financing. To implement its policies the board of a hospital appoints medical staff, an administrator, and certain other personnel. The Board's responsibilities are set out in provincial statutes, and regulations governing public hospitals. In Ontario, for example, Regulation 523 under the Public Hospitals Act specifies that " ... a hospital shall be governed and managed by a board elected or appointed in accordance with the provisions of the authority under which the hospital is created, established or incorporated."[5] Under this Act the Board is responsible for passing by-laws that govern "the appointment and functioning of (i) an administrator or superintendent, (ii) a medical staff, and (iii) a person licensed under the *Public Accountancy Act* as an auditor."[6]

The governing body is the ultimate source of authority in the hospital,

2 / *Ibid.*, p. 20.

3 / Robert N. Wilson, "The Social Structure of a General Hospital," *Annals of the American Academy of Political and Social Science*, vol. 346, March 1963, p. 68.

4 / *Ibid.*

5 / The Public Hospitals Act, R.R.O., 1960, Reg. 523, s.2.

6 / The Public Hospitals Act, R.R.O., 1960, Reg. 523, s.6.

but since the introduction of the Hospital Insurance and Diagnostic Services Act in Canada, this authority has been attenuated in certain hospitals to some extent, mainly because provincial governments, which have the constitutional responsibility under the British North America Act for health matters, have sought to rationalize individual hospital operations by stressing an increasing degree of budgetary accountability on the part of the hospitals. In Ontario the Hospital Services Commission requires each hospital in the province to submit its financial requirements for approval by the Commission prior to the beginning of each fiscal year. The requirement enables the Commission to revise and sometimes eliminate certain budgetary items. This type of financial control sometimes restricts the authority of the governing body, whose members may feel that the independence of their institution, which in many cases was founded through community effort, is being curtailed.

Some indication of the reaction of hospital officials to this erosion of independence is evident in the briefs of provincial hospital associations presented to the Royal Commission on Health Services; for example, the brief submitted to the Commission by the Associated Hospitals of Alberta includes as an appendix a brief submitted to the Minister of Health of that province in 1962. The appendix states that use of hospitals is growing, and requires an increase both qualitatively and quantitatively in hospital personnel. Provincial government officials seeking to control the rate of growth of hospital expenditures, laid down procedures whose purpose was to eliminate "over use" but these, according to this source, denied services to patients needing them. As the appendix states:

Medical procedures are of little value unless they are used. Those who can benefit from such procedures will demand that they are used promptly and effectively. Hospitals and doctors have no alternative except to make such procedures immediately available. It is highly unfair for hospitals and their medical staffs, as a consequence of such increased use and increased costs, to be charged with over-use and to have their costs disallowed. The only alternative is an effect on the welfare of the community in terms of the quality and quantity of patient services which are available to the sick and injured.[7]

In the preamble to the recommendations contained in the brief of the Associated Hospitals of Alberta to the Minister of Health of that province the following statement appears which indicates that a government's insistence on economic rationality in hospital operations has aroused fears of government control on the part of hospital authorities.

7 / Associated Hospitals of Alberta, *Brief Submitted to the Royal Commission on Health Services*, Edmonton: February 1962, Appendix II, p. 5.

The member hospitals of the Associated Hospitals of Alberta are desirous of providing service for the people of their respective communities which is adequate both as to quality and quantity. They feel sure that you share this desire with them, but fear that serious misunderstandings are developing concerning hospital economics which threaten to weaken the effectiveness of the hospital insurance plan as the principal means of financing hospital care in the province. They, and no doubt you, are anxious to avoid such an occurrence.[8]

Within the hospital, the administrator or superintendent is responsible to the board for implementing its policies by co-ordinating the activities of hospital personnel directed towards the goal of patient treatment. In some hospitals the administrative function will be the responsibility of a lay person and the medical function will be the responsibility of a physician with both officers reporting to the governing body through a joint advisory committee. In his administrative and co-ordinating function an administrator is guided by the policies or intentions of the board. He is responsible for preparing the hospital budget for approval by the board and within the limitations imposed by the budget he is expected to employ or discharge personnel and to fix salary scales; to maintain liaison between the board, and members of the medical staff of clinical departments including clinical department heads; to see that the professional orders of physicians practising in the hospital are carried out by hospital staff; and to formulate detailed regulations for the operation of the hospital.

The medical function is delegated by the board to the medical staff which includes those physicians practising in the community in which the hospital is located who have been appointed to the medical staff of the hospital by the Board through the recommendation of the medical staff of the hospital. This function is performed by clinical departments representing a range of specialties such as medicine, surgery, obstetrics, gynaecology, dermatology, urology, ophthalmology, radiology, and others. Each clinical department is led by a department head to whom the board, through the administrator, delegates responsibility for the provision of medical care under professional controls according to specified standards. In teaching hospitals the department head is also responsible for the education of medical students, interns, and residents. Although the board is responsible for policy in matters relating to the medical treatment of patients, it does not originate it. This responsibility is delegated to the medical staff which has a number of committees such as a tissue committee, a medical records committee, a credentials committee, a medical audit committee, and a pharmacy committee. In its area of concern each of these committees initiates and implements policies concerning standards

8 / *Ibid.,* p. 14.

and procedures affecting medical treatment.[9]

On the surface the formal organization of the hospital apparently resembles Weber's model of a fully rationalized bureaucracy in which the officials are appointed on the basis of technical competence to a hierarchy of offices graded according to their level of authority and bound by rules which govern the actions of their incumbents. The office holder in the hospital does not own the things with which he works, in many cases he is remunerated by a fixed salary scale within a formal promotional system, and is limited in the exercise of authority by the sphere of the authority of the office he holds.

The hospital has certain goals, and like other bureaucracies where large numbers of people are organized for particular purposes, these ends cannot be assured with any degree of certainty unless those who are organized behave in a predictable fashion. Predictability of human behaviour is one of the chief purposes of a bureaucracy, although the degree of predictability may vary from one bureaucracy to another depending upon the severity of the strains and conflicts generated within the organization in the attempt to bring individuals of diverse social backgrounds together to act in specified ways, at specified times, and for specified purposes. In order to bring the available knowledge and techniques to bear on particular cases of illness, individuals possessing different skills must be brought to a case at particular times and in specified places, to carry out their specially skilled activities. Time, place, and skill must be made available and it is the purpose of the collective rules to assure their availability.

THE PHYSICIAN IN THE HOSPITAL HIERARCHY

The governing body of a hospital is composed of people who are generally persons of high business or professional standing with influence in their community. These individuals tend to reflect the social and political climate of the community they serve and are not radically different from it.[10] The board can appoint physicians to the hospital staff, but it lacks the technical competence to control the day-to-day activities of the physician in the hospital. In the diagnosis and treatment of his patient's ills, the physician has the ultimate authority which is based on his professional technical competence, but his conception of what is best for his patient may conflict with the policies laid down by the board. However, unlike that of most hospital administrators, the physicians' social background is

9 / For a brief description of the work of these Committees see p. 78.
10 / Temple E. Burling *et al.*, *The Give and Take in Hospitals*, New York: G. P. Putnam's Sons, 1956, p. 37.

generally similar to that of the board members; they have usually attended the same schools, have similar attitudes and tastes and mix with one another on social occasions; these similarities produce a likeness of perspective which can help the board members and physicians to bridge the misunderstandings which may separate them in the hospital.

The office of administrator is relatively new in hospital organization. The increased demand for this type of official could not be met from the ranks of the medical or nursing profession although representatives of both have been trained to perform this role. It was met initially by training accounting and clerical personnel in administrative skills through a combination of correspondence courses and on-the-job training. With the emergence of hospital administration as a recognized skill, more formal training and educational programmes were organized in universities. But a training in administrative skills gives the student administrator only a meagre understanding of the world of medicine. This lack of understanding of technical medical matters on the part of the administrator tends to create conflict between him and the physician practising in the hospital. Furthermore, the social distance between the two groups, manifested in different social perspectives and values, provides a fertile seed bed in which misunderstanding can flourish.

With the centralization of the technology of medical care in the hospital, the organization of this institution grew more complex. As noted earlier, in order to bring the available medical knowledge and technology to bear on particular cases of illness, individuals possessing different skills must apply them in the diagnosis and treatment of particular cases at a specified time and place, and an organizational structure is required to meet this purpose. The role of the hospital administrator is to see that this structure operates to meet this end. He symbolizes the bureaucratic element in hospital organization whereas the physician symbolizes the professional and technical element. The administrator sees the hospital as having an institutional mission of its own, as being "able to undertake some of the things that doctors cannot do, either as individuals or as a group. Although there is no doubt that the hospital provides 'hospital care' it is not always clear just where hospital care ends and medical care begins."[11] On the other hand, for the physician the hospital is a public utility which he can use for professional purposes, the treatment of his patients; for him this is the main, if not the sole, function of the institution. That there should be a difference in the conception of the goal of the hospital held by administrators and physicians is due to the lack of specificity of the institution's goals.

11 / Richard M. Magraw and Daniel B. Magraw, *Ferment in Medicine*, Philadelphia: W. B. Saunders Co., 1966, p. 106.

Most medical institutions are concerned with promoting health and preventing illness, but who has yet satisfactorily defined these states? ... lack of specificity of objectives will reverberate throughout the structure as disagreements over choosing tasks to be performed, personnel to be hired, resources to be allocated, members to be compensated and status and authority to be distributed.[12]

These differences between physician and hospital administrator are further exacerbated by the authority system of the hospital which gives the administrator, as the representative of the board, the responsibility for the care of the patient although the actual treatment of the patient is prescribed by the physician. In effect the administrator is responsible to the board for seeing that its policies are carried out by the medical staff. On the other hand, the medical staff of the hospital is responsible for actually providing medical care of an accepted standard according to the judgment of medical peers, and for a high degree of self-regulation and control through various committees of peers who judge the quality of an individual physician's work. This highly professionalized group, with long-standing traditions of service, professional autonomy, technical competence, and self-regulation must nevertheless obey the dictates of the administrator whose administrative authority exceeds that of the hospital physician.

One reason for the greater administrative authority of the hospital administrator relative to the hospital physician is that the institution is a public utility to serve the health needs of the community. As noted earlier, with the introduction of the Hospital Insurance and Diagnostic Services Act in Canada the extent of provincial government control of hospital administration and financing has substantially increased.[13] The hospital board is the representative of the community and its elected politicians and the hospital administrator is directly responsible to the board for the day-to-day operation of this public utility. The physician, therefore, does not own or control the institution although he cannot practise effectively without it. Furthermore, although his earnings depend to a large extent on the use he makes of hospital equipment, services, and facilities he does not pay for their use. His authority is restricted to technical medical matters. He is a guest in the institution, and he must bow to the ultimate authority of the board and to the administrative authority of its representative. A severe strain is placed upon the physician when his professional authority, based upon his technical competence, conflicts with that of the administrator who through the board controls the physician's access to and use of the technical equipment and services he requires to perform

12 / W. Richard Scott, *Some Implications of Organization Theory for Research on Health Services*, United States Public Health Services, New York: 1966, p. 40.
13 / See p. 71.

this professional role and thereby earn a living. It is this conflict between two lines of authority which is the genesis of much of the strain the physician faces as he practises in the hospital.

Within the hospital the myriad of specialized activities can only be directed to the goal of the institution, the care of the patient, if these activities are co-ordinated, and co-ordination can only be realized through a functioning hierarchy of authority. In Simon's words, "procedural co-ordination establishes the lines of authority and outlines the spheres of activity of each organization member, while substantive coordination specifies the content of his work."[14] Within the hospital, then, procedural co-ordination is brought about through the use of administrative authority, whereas substantive co-ordination is the result of the use of professional authority. It is obvious that in the contemporary hospital, where technical change and development are proceeding at a pace probably unmatched by any other social institution, or indeed in the history of this particular institution, confusion and overlapping in the use of authority, administrative or professional, are almost inevitable. That this situation creates strains in the role of the physician, therefore, should not be unexpected.

At heart, the hospital is more like a federal system than a monolithic entity; its organization takes the form of a federation of departments, each department enjoying considerable autonomy and discretion in its management of work. The great challenge is, then, one of coordination, of somehow knitting these special excellences into a comprehensive framework of care. We have seen that the patient, by his very presence, is a coordinating force. But the needs of the ill are not enough and are today progressively supplemented by the shaping patterns of rational bureaucracy.[15]

In the day-to-day operations of the hospitals, then, the two lines of authority, one of which directs the medical and the other the administrative activity, can overlap. But such conflicts of interest between physicians and administrators seem to emerge as an inherent characteristic of the modern hospital which embraces the independent and professionally autonomous physician seeking to apply his skills for the treatment of patients for whose medical welfare he is ultimately responsible, and the administrator whose co-ordinating function requires him to direct the activities of the physician. "Clashes between administrative and medical desiderata are among the most disruptive of hospital conflicts; [and] they are truly structural and thus only very partially dependent on the personal idiosyncracies of specific doctors or administrators."[16]

14 / Herbert A. Simon, *Administrative Behaviour*, 2nd ed., New York: The Macmillan Co., 1958, p. 10.

15 / Wilson, "The Social Structure of a General Hospital," p. 74.

16 / *Ibid.*, p. 71.

Besides the strains facing the hospital physician stemming from the conflict between professional and administrative authority, he encounters other difficulties in his professional role in the hospital. These emerge out of the conflict between different levels of professional medical authority where one level seeks to control the activities of another. Control by colleagues of their members' activities is the hallmark of a profession, the authority for such control being delegated to the profession by the state, and exercised by a licensing and disciplinary body organized by the profession. Control of day-to-day professional activities is, in the first instance, the responsibility of the individual professional, whom the professional body trusts to act in the prescribed professional manner so that his client's interests and welfare are safeguarded. That this trust may sometimes be misplaced may not be due to lack of professional ethics on the part of the professional so much as to the strains imposed on him by the changing context in which he works. The physician attempts to play out his professional role in the medical market place where he faces a rising demand for care from an increasingly sophisticated public critical of the greater costs of care but insisting that it be of the highest standard. This situation of increasing demand and costs requires the application of new and old medical knowledge in new ways and in new organizational forms so that demand can be met in the most economically efficient manner.

The responsibility for the professional activities of the physician practising in the hospital lies with the hospital's medical advisory committee and its supporting committees. The extent to which these committees effectively discharge their responsibilities may sometimes be open to question, but their existence creates an awareness in the practitioner that his professional activities can be scrutinized and judged by his peers. Without such a scrutiny mistakes could become more frequent and the quality of medical care deteriorate with the result that the public would eventually realize the danger it faces with a consequent damage to the image of the profession.

That the medical profession is aware of the role of the medical advisory committee in maintaining the quality of medical care in the hospital is evident from recent discussions in various professional medical journals. Williams and Osbaldeston, for example, state that:

The concept that physicians, especially those in the hospital setting, must be their brother's keeper is not a new one. A basic principle of the Canadian Council on Hospital Accreditation states that the medical staff of a hospital must accept responsibility for the professional practices of its members.... Intraprofessional guidance and stimulus are largely responsible for the high calibre of hospital practice in Canada and the United States today, even though some hospital medical staffs may fail to recognize fully their continuing responsibility to maintain the present high standards.[17]

In its supervision of the professional activities of the hospital medical staff, the medical advisory committee is assisted by a number of other committees. A direct control of the quality of medical care in hospitals may be exercised by the credentials committee which scrutinizes the qualifications and experience of those physicians seeking to practise in the hospital, and specifies the type of professional activities which they are allowed to undertake in the institution. Tissue committees study the tissues removed by surgeons to determine if their removal was warranted. Medical audit committees "review medical records, pre- and post-operative diagnoses and other measures, and provide a standard method of evaluation of the medical care provided by physicians."[18] Medical records committees "study the quality of the physician's records of his patient and establish an acceptable standard."[19] A recent innovation in the control of medical practice in the hospital is the Professional Activity Study. In this type of study medical data are obtained from the medical records of the hospital for the purpose of reviewing the clinical work of the physician and undertaking special clinical studies. Such a study "makes it possible for a medical staff to obtain a view of medical practice not previously accessible. Specific entities may be selected for a detailed audit, or comparisons may be drawn with other hospitals."[20]

In those hospitals where these committees are organized the fact of their existence exercises a pressure upon the physician to live up to standards. Nevertheless, as Clute points out with respect to general practice, and as the concern of the medical profession regarding the quality of care suggests, these controls may not be completely effective.

Despite the importance of the medical advisory committee with respect to the quality of medical care there is no such body in some hospitals, particularly small hospitals. In Ontario, for example, privileges for hospital use have been granted to physicians without a study or investigation of their credentials, and surgeons have been allowed to undertake "very major procedures in a small hospital lacking in the physical facilities and technical and ancillary personnel considered necessary for the safety and

17 / K. J. Williams and J. B. Osbaldeston, "The Hospital Medical Advisory Committee: The Cabinet of the Medical Staff," *Canadian Medical Association Journal*, vol. 92, May 22, 1965, p. 1117.

18 / J. A. MacFarlane, *Medical Education in Canada*, Royal Commission on Health Services, Ottawa: Queen's Printer, 1964, p. 277.

19 / *Ibid.*

20 / Williams and Osbaldeston, "The Hospital Advisory Committee," p. 1121.

welfare of the patient."[21] Even in large hospitals "laxity has been known to occur and privileges have been granted, or allowed to continue in effect, in the case of practitioners whose knowledge, skill or professional conduct left something to be desired."[22] In Ontario, this situation, in fact, is due to the present statutory provisions which do not give senior physicians in the hospital, such as chiefs of staff and heads of departments, the authority to intervene in the treatment of the patient. The Public Hospitals Act of Ontario does not give this authority even when the senior medical staff see that its use is required.[23]

The extent and nature of the limitations on medical staff privileges in Canada may be similar to the experience in the United States. If Michigan can be taken as an example of that experience, a study of controls in hospitals revealed that 70 per cent of hospitals with 500 or more beds had some restrictions on privileges in six areas of practice compared with 47 per cent of hospitals with 100 to 499 beds, and only 26 per cent in small hospitals of less than 100 beds.[24] In effect, the quality of medical care deteriorates as the size of the hospital decreases. Lacking comparable data it is difficult to determine the extent to which this holds true in Canada. Nevertheless, as Dawson indicates, the small hospital faces serious obstacles to the control of quality through restrictions on the granting of privileges.[25] He points out, however, that in Ontario, despite these obstacles, "in 50% of small hospitals full privileges will be granted to an applicant who submits a current annual certificate of registration issued by the College of Physicians and Surgeons of Ontario."[26]

In limiting the hospital privileges of a physician the medical advisory committee, in effect, is limiting his earning power for he must refer to colleagues those patients requiring services which he is not permitted to perform. Such a limitation becomes a restriction on the status and prestige of the physician when his peers evaluate his competence in relation to those who are given wider privileges. Competition for status, therefore, becomes a matter of professional control of patients. Even a highly qualified specialist may be required to limit his skills to his recognized area of competence.

---

21 / J. C. C. Dawson, "The Quality of Medical Care – A Joint Responsibility," *Report of the College of Physicians and Surgeons of Ontario*, January 1965, p. 24.
22 / *Ibid.*, p. 23.
23 / *Ibid.*, p. 25.
24 / Walter J. McNerney, *Hospital and Medical Economics*, vol. 2, Chicago: Hospital Research and Educational Trusts, 1962, pp. 1232–33.
25 / Dawson, "Quality of Care," p. 25.
26 / *Ibid.*, p. 26.

In hospitals where privileges have been defined such competition is limited to other facets of the physician's role, with the specialist usually having more prestige than the general practitioner and, within specialties, the surgeon more than the obstetrician. Moreover, within the medical profession, as within other professions, there exists generally a struggle for prestige and the symbols of prestige such as degrees, institutional affiliations, membership in learned societies, publications and so on, with the winner in the struggle gaining greater confidence from the public and assurance of a demand for his services which may increase in cost as his prestige rises.

The foregoing analysis has provided some indication of the genesis of two major types of role strain facing a physician practising in the hospital; strains which are generated by the conflict between two types of authority, the professional and the administrative, and by the conflict among physicians in their attempt to maintain standards of quality. There is yet another type of role strain which a physician encounters in a hospital. This is related to the increasing number and complexity of the nursing and paramedical personnel employed by that institution.

The independent practitioner, accustomed to a purely private relationship with his patient and to absolute authority over auxiliary personnel when he came to the hospital has joined a medical "team." Former aides have grown into full-fledged collaborators. His once unquestioned monopoly of professional status increasingly gives way to the claims of nurse, hospital administrator, social worker, dietitian, physical therapist, and others.[27]

Hospitals seem to generate the professionalization of the special paramedical skills to which they gave birth such as those of the nurse, the laboratory technician, the x-ray technician, the operating room technician, the medical record librarian, the electroencephalographer and others. These skills have emerged within the hospital and grown with it for it is in the hospital that the technology, the technical equipment, the laboratory, the occupational therapy equipment, the operating rooms, and the patients are, in the main, located. If the services which this equipment provides are to be given to patients, these paramedical personnel must become part of the hospital. Their skills are nurtured by the hospital setting and are increasingly bound to it.

The cost of the technical equipment operated by paramedical personnel has prevented private ownership by physicians or technicians. Collective ownership through public financing is the accepted means of obtaining it. Furthermore, the services provided by this equipment are interdependent;

27 / Samuel W. Bloom, *The Doctor and His Patient*, New York: Russell Sage Foundation, 1963, p. 161.

they provide the physician with a comprehensive diagnostic picture or a set of interrelated therapeutic aids. Quick access to these services, in many cases, is of paramount importance in saving life. For reasons of cost, complexity, and availability, therefore, this equipment has been centrally located in the hospital. Thus, the tools which the technician must use are a public utility forcing him to depend upon the public as represented by the hospital board for the practice of his skills. He can only practise these skills by accepting the authority of the collectivity as represented by the hospital administrator for it is this authority which provides him with a place to work and the tools of his trade. Without these he cannot function. However, each of these paramedical groups depends upon the physician practising in the hospital for the initiation of orders which call his or her special skills into play. This dependence creates tensions within the hospital for, in spite of this dependence, these groups are striving for professional status, and its accompanying psychic rewards.

Although these paramedical personnel are subject to the authority of the physician with a hospital appointment, and to the authority of the hospital board which is delegated to the hospital administrator, they do exert some control over the hospital physician. In order to provide an acceptable standard of care he must depend on the skill of these groups and this dependence gives the paramedical group a degree of control over the manner in which medicine is practised. The physician can no longer practise in true solo fashion in the hospital. His dependence on others, a dependence that will undoubtedly increase as medical technology grows even more complex, conflicts with the accepted professional notions of independence and autonomy which he has learned initially in medical school and later during his hospital training. Dependence on others striving to professionalize their skills and competing for prestige may pose threats to the physician's status. This may best be illustrated by a discussion of the changing role and status of the nurse.

The current public view of the hospital as a place of treatment and care rather than custody, the growth of medical technology centralized in the hospital, the increased demand for hospital care, and the emergence of the hospital as the physician's workshop have resulted in a growing demand for nursing skills in that institution. These developments have been accompanied by a desire for professional status by nurses based, in part at least, on the gradual transference to the nurse of a number of technical medical procedures hitherto the responsibility of the physician. This transfer has resulted, in turn, in the delegating of certain nursing responsibilities to subordinates, including those activities which nurses find disagreeable. As Hall says, "... there are some activities which are almost revoltingly disagreeable to the members concerned. When an occasion arises, these are relegated to a lower class of worker who, for the time being, find the work passably agreeable."[28] By relegating these activities to subordinates, the nurse has been able to focus her attention on administrative and teaching functions.

She is responsible for the management of a team of personnel under her authority: student nurses, practical nurses, and aides. Her duties have become specialized both in the fact that she has had to assume managerial functions on the ward and floor, and in the fact that her nursing has become focused upon a specialty (obstetrics, pediatrics, surgical, etc.). The diffuse and generalized responsibilities of the nurse, as they have been traditionally defined, no longer are valid characterizations of her present duties and functions.[29]

Some nurses, however, seem unwilling to accept new responsibilities since it means delegating to others old responsibilities from which they gain emotional satisfaction. This reluctance is evident in their opposition to reforms in nursing education which attempt to change traditional nursing values and socialize students into a conception of the new nursing role. For those who support these reforms, these changes not only bring nursing into touch with the realities of twentieth-century medicine, but they also mean a change in the status of the nurse. In other words, this occupation, like medicine and a host of others, is engaged in a struggle for status and prestige which becomes particularly severe as new occupations and professions emerge. These new fields of endeavour, being based on the findings of modern science, have substantial prestige in the eyes of the public, and they offer to those in the process of making an occupational choice alternatives to the older occupations and professions. Nursing must successfully compete for status and prestige with this growing list of alternative occupations.

Since the introduction of the first training school for nurses in Canada nursing education for the great majority has been undertaken by hospitals. Under this system, students were given training in exchange for services to the hospital, but these services took precedence over educational and training requirements.[30] As the responsibilities of nurses changed, the demand for more highly skilled practitioners increased. Universities attempted to meet this demand by setting up programmes of nursing education. Today the profession is demanding that the nursing education

28 / Oswald Hall, "Specialized Occupations and Industrial Unrest," lecture delivered at Tulane University, 1957.

29 / Leonard Reissman and John H. Rohrer, *Change and Dilemma in the Nursing Profession*, New York: G. P. Putnam's Sons, 1957, p. 13.

30 / Helen K. Mussallem, *Nursing Education in Canada*, Royal Commission on Health Services, Ottawa: Queen's Printer, 1965, p. 6.

function of the hospital be taken over by educational bodies, and that the distinction between nurses trained in hospital schools of nursing and those completing a university degree in nursing be rationalized on the basis of a division of labour between the two groups.

The role to be assumed by the professional nurse implies that she should have a professional education as a basis for developing a high level of professional and technical competence. This competence can be developed only if the practitioner has a sound understanding of scientific principles, as contrasted to the applied science which would be the basis for operation of the technical nurse.[31]

Efforts are now underway in Saskatchewan to transfer the responsibility for the training of nurses from hospitals to educational authorities. In Ontario, educational standards are set by the Ontario College of Nursing with the Hospital Services Commission providing the hospital with a separate budget for nursing education which is the responsibility of the Director of Nursing Education. This is probably an interim step before the function is made the responsibility of educational authorities.

These changes in the nursing role, supported by changes in educational preparation and in licensing arrangements, affect the relationship between physician and nurse. For the physician, these developments pose a competitive threat to his status, but nurses are only one of an increasing number of paramedical occupations in hospitals seeking to further their professional status through the symbolic accoutrements of university courses, professional associations with licensing powers, and sometimes the actual treatment of patients.

Thus the hospital is not only caught up in rapid technical change, but change in its social organization as well, with nurses and other paramedical personnel seeking to raise their professional standing and competing for prestige. In order to practise modern medicine, the physician must rely upon the services of nurses and the paramedical group, some of whom have to operate the highly technical equipment of the hospital. These innovations in technology could have had a much different "feed back" effect on the organization of medical care if they had not been located mainly in the hospital. For reasons stated earlier, they were concentrated in the hospital, thus leaving the form of medical practice outside that institution more or less in its traditional form. The physician in solo practice, for example, is still able to invest in an office and the necessary but limited tools of his trade while maintaining a close relationship with the hospital and control over the treatment of his hospitalized patients. But in his association with a hospital, he leaves himself open to the demands for

31 / *Ibid.*, p. 123.

status and prestige of the administrators, and professional technicians required to operate the complex hospital apparatus. The hospital has become a seed bed of professionalization and the physician is now placed in a position where he must constantly seek to protect his status.

Not only must he seek to protect himself from the professional encroachments of those occupations generated by the division of labour within the hospital, but he must also face another threat from other professions in the community seeking to apply their skills in the hospital. These professions, such as social work and dentistry, have developed in the community to serve clients. They have, more or less, the recognized professional criteria and those engaged in them are accepted by the public as professional persons. These groups are now demanding that they be allowed to follow their clients into the hospital, there to apply their skills and be recognized as professional persons on the "medical team." For these groups the hospital functions as an additional context in which their skills may be applied. The physician, on the other hand, recognizing this development as another threat to his authority in the hospital, seeks to ensure that his status there is undiminished by maintaining the inviolability of the medical authority system and thus placing the newcomers in the difficult position of either accepting the dominance of the administrative authority or of attempting to follow the pattern set by the physicians.

6

THE SELF-GOVERNING
PROFESSION

THE PRECEDING CHAPTERS have indicated the manner in which a physician, as he goes about his day-to-day practice whether in his office, a patient's home, or a hospital is controlled to a greater or less extent by the formal and informal sanctions of professional colleagues and other health personnel. The range of these controls and the degree to which they actually influence the physician's behaviour depend, to a significant extent, as we have seen, on the institutional context in which the physician applies his skills. Controls on his professional behaviour are also applied by professional organizations, of which the two most important, at the provincial level, are the College of Physicians and Surgeons, and the provincial division of the Canadian Medical Association. Each of these two provincial bodies is represented in the corresponding national organizations, the Royal College of Physicians and Surgeons of Canada and the Canadian Medical Association. These organizations lay down the norms which are intended to govern professional behaviour, and in general they seek to protect the status and economic security of their members and to raise standards of professional performance.

THE PROVINCIAL COLLEGE OF PHYSICIANS AND SURGEONS

Since matters pertaining to health and education are a constitutional responsibility of each of the Canadian provinces, each College of Physicians and Surgeons is incorporated under a provincial act. The intent of these acts is twofold: "first, to protect the public by prescribing the qualifications for practitioners, licensing annually those so qualified, and providing penalties for those who violate the standards or practise medicine without being licensed; second, to delegate the responsibility of administering the act to those to whom it applies."[1]

1 / Malcolm G. Taylor, "The Role of the Medical Profession in the Formulation and Execution of Public Policy," *Canadian Journal of Economics and Political Science*, vol. 26, February 1960, p. 110.

The policy of a provincial college is the responsibility of a council of elected or appointed college members. In Ontario, for example, the council consists of "A twelve physicians elected from the ten territorial divisions in Ontario – three of whom will be from Metropolitan Toronto; B one member to be appointed by each of the four medical faculties in Ontario; c The Minister of Health of the Province of Ontario."[2] Other than the four members appointed by the universities in the province with a medical school, academic physicians are specifically excluded from membership on the Council.[3]

The Medical Act in each province requires the College to maintain a register of all those who have met the basic requirements for the practice of medicine, which are specified in the Act and include the necessary educational qualifications. The specifications of these qualifications vary between provinces, but the powers of the College may include the right to set the final year examinations and the curriculum of the medical school. This statutory power to prescribe the curriculum of studies to be pursued by medical students could be used to control curriculum in medical schools and the professional orientation of their graduates. The exercise of this type of control could in turn affect the institutional development of medical practice. However, the Ontario College claims that "Whenever major changes in the curriculum are contemplated, the universities in Ontario consult the College through their representative on the Council or by consultation between the College and the Deans of the Faculties of Medicine."[4]

Social and economic changes may create pressures for change in the physician's role which could result in changes in the social organization of practice, but the statutory power to determine both the technical and the cultural content of the role, which lies with the College of Physicians and Surgeons at the provincial level and the Royal College of Physicians and Surgeons at the national level, is sufficient to resist such pressures for change. On the other hand this power could be used to create new patterns of medical education and of medical practice which are more closely integrated with the social structure of twentieth-century Canada. The present lack of integration is reflected in the role strains of the physician. Its historical antecedents may be identified in the recommendations of the *Flexner Report*, referred to in chapter 3, which resulted in the creation of a uniform type of medical school in which the first two years of instruction emphasized the basic sciences and the final two years concentrated on

2 / College of Physicians and Surgeons of Ontario, *Brief Submitted to the Royal Commission on Health Services*, Toronto: May 1962, Appendix 14, p. 6.
3 / The Medical Act, R.S.O., 1960, chapter 234, section 3.
4 / College of Physicians and Surgeons of Ontario, *Brief Submitted to the Ontario Committee on the Healing Arts*, part 1, Toronto: July 1967, p. 4.

clinical training; the raising of educational standards in medical schools in Canada and the United States; and improvement in the quality of medical care. The Report, however, was written in an era when medical knowledge and technology were in an almost rudimentary state compared with today. Furthermore, the society of Flexner's era had yet to undergo the many fundamental social changes which are now evident. Nevertheless, the Report is still enshrined as the *raison d'être* for many aspects of the present organization of medical education and licensing which were its consequences.

There is, however, a concern on the part of some segments of the medical profession, more particularly medical educators, with the lack of integration between medicine and other social institutions. For medical educators in both Canada and the United States the institutional resistance to change is the result of a "discontinuity" in medical education. "Responsibility in medical education is shared by the universities, medical schools, hospitals and professional organizations. And this arrangement, which creates a 'discontinuity' in medical education, also accounts for medicine's deficiency in planning and policy-making."[5]

The provincial colleges are given the power to erase from the register the names of all those who are convicted for certain offences under the law although the physician concerned can appeal such decisions. In Ontario this type of disciplinary control is a funtcion of the Council of the College; its decisions may be appealed to the Appeal Court of Ontario but they have usually been upheld by the courts. "The courts have repeatedly held that what constitutes this sort of professional conduct by a licensed practitioner is properly the judgement, after a fair hearing by his peers, i.e., the Council of the College."[6] According to College spokesmen, "We are of the opinion that this is right and that fair-minded members of the profession are the only groups qualified to decide what is and what is not proper conduct of a member of the medical profession and no change is necessary or advised in this matter."[7]

Nevertheless, Mr. Justice James McRuer in the report of his Inquiry into Civil Rights in Ontario states that there are dangers in the operation of what are essentially private courts:

Disciplinary powers are penal powers. When these powers are conferred on private individuals who take no oath of office, and for whom in most cases the government has no responsibility for appointment, a private court is created ...

5 / Commonwealth Fund and Carnegie Corporation of New York, *The Crisis in Medical Services and Medical Education*, Report on an Exploratory Conference, Florida: 1966, p. 7.
6 / College of Physicians and Surgeons of Ontario, *Brief Submitted to the Royal Commission on Health Services*, p. 3.
7 / *Ibid.*

In general, questions of professional or occupational misconduct, incompetence and unethical practices are matters which the leading members of a profession or occupation should be best able to judge. However, the ability born of experience to decide what is and what is not professional or occupational misconduct, is not necessarily the same thing as the ability to occupy satisfactorily the seat of justice. There is in the present situation a very real danger that the protection of public, professional and occupational interests will cause the other interests involved to be disregarded.

The practitioner against whom disciplinary proceedings are directed has a very real interest in the fairness of the proceedings. Basic concepts of penal justice, such as the presumption of innocence, have just as much place in such proceedings as in the courts of law. Unless the interests and rights of the accused are protected under the present system, or unless the present system can be modified by the introduction of safe-guards for those interests and rights, the argument is very strong that the right to dispense private professional penal justice should be withdrawn and all disciplinary matters be decided by the courts of law.[8]

The practising physician today must cope with a medical and non-medical environment in which the application of his skills is made more and more difficult as both these interacting contexts change at an increasing rate. This difficulty creates a growing possibility of error and sanctions by his professional peers. In Ontario the most common reasons for consideration of sanctions are negligence or any act of professional misconduct, criminal offences committed in the practice of medicine, incompetence in hospital practice, mishandling of drugs on the Narcotic or Controlled Drug List, violation of the code of ethics, and fraud in the handling of claims from insuring agencies.[9] Whether the growing possibility of error and ineptitude has resulted in an increase in their occurrence cannot be determined with available data, but Clute in Canada and Peterson in the United States have indicated clearly that error and ineptitude exist.[10] Recognition by laymen that they do exist is prevented to some extent by professional norms regarding public evaluation by professionals of colleagues' behaviour, and by public ignorance of professional matters. The public must depend on the professional body to protect it from medical error and ineptitude, a responsibility which has been delegated to

8 / Ontario, Royal Commission Inquiry into Civil Rights, *Report no. 1*, vol. 3, Toronto: Queen's Printer, 1968, pp. 1182–83.

9 / College of Physicians and Surgeons of Ontario, "Answers to Questionnaire 'A' for Submission to the Province of Ontario, Committee on the Healing Arts," 1966.

10 / K. F. Clute, *The General Practitioner*, Toronto: University of Toronto Press, 1963, and Osler L. Peterson *et al.*, "An Analytical Study of North Carolina General Practice, 1953–1954," *Journal of Medical Education*, vol. 31, no. 12, December 1956, part 2.

the profession by statute. In discharging this responsibility the profession must protect both the public and the profession. Failure to do the latter, as Goode points out, would "create a Hobbesian jungle, the undermining of group structure, the loss of the usual benefits of organization and cooperation, and the dissolution of group loyalties."[11]

The Ontario College also wishes to widen its powers to include some control of the licensing of paramedical personnel such as registered nurses, laboratory and x-ray technicians, occupational therapists and physiotherapists, psychologists and others. "The education, qualifications and integrity of these auxiliaries should be governed by a licensing body and since their work is so closely associated with that of the registered doctors this should possibly be through, or by association with, the College."[12] Such a development could give the College a supervisory power over the professional bodies representing these paramedical personnel and provide it with "an opportunity to protect its competitive interests as opposed to the interests of the members of the public."[13]

Through the power granted by government to this type of professional association at the provincial level, the profession is assured of a degree of self-government and independence probably greater than in any other profession, a power that reaches out to control, directly or indirectly, the activities of other recognized professional groups, and also educational qualifications and standards; even universities, traditionally jealous of their autonomy as centres of learning and research, must legally conform to the educational dictates of the College.

The economic security of a physician depends to an important degree on the demand for his services and the supply of qualified physicians to meet it. If supply does not expand to meet demand, the physician's income may rise, but his work-load will probably increase. In Canada in recent years existing medical schools have been enlarged to accommodate additional students, new medical schools have been built, and the provincial colleges have licensed large numbers of immigrant physicians. These developments have increased the supply of physicians. Nevertheless, it is apparent that demand still exceeds the capacity to meet it. Part of the necessary increase in supply could be met by increasing the number of qualified alien physicians licensed to practise in Canada, but evidence suggests that the licensing power of the colleges of physicians and surgeons has

11 / William J. Goode, "The Protection of the Inept," *American Sociological Review*, vol. 32, no. 1, February 1967, p. 15.

12 / College of Physicians and Surgeons of Ontario, *Brief Submitted to the Royal Commission on Health Services*, p. 4.

13 / Ontario, Royal Commission Inquiry into Civil Rights, *Report Number One*, vol. 3, p. 1204.

been used to limit the number of licensed alien physicians. The usual reason given for this restriction is that the standards of medical education in the country in which the alien completed his medical education are lower than the standards of medical education in Canada. Nevertheless, each provincial licensing body attempts to assess these foreign standards in its own way with the result that there is a lack of uniformity between provinces in the assessment of foreign standards.

Physicians seeking to practise in Canada who are registered on the "General List" of the General Medical Council of Great Britain can register by reciprocal arrangement without further examination in Alberta, Saskatchewan, Manitoba, Nova Scotia, Prince Edward Island, and Newfoundland. This reciprocal arrangement is used by many of these immigrating physicians as a means of gaining entry into the profession in Canada; they then seek a practice in a location of their choice. In Nova Scotia, for example, "... in 1961, of 34 registering by reciprocity only 9 entered practice in Nova Scotia."[14]

For the graduates of foreign medical schools who are not registered on the "General List" of the General Medical Council of Great Britain, the obstacles to be overcome before they can practise in Canada are indeed discouraging. They must pass examinations set by the provincial licensing authority, "which include usually such subjects as anatomy, biochemistry, physiology, pathology, bacteriology and pharmacology,"[15] although there is some variation between provinces in these requirements. They must also complete "one or two years of satisfactory rotating internship in a hospital located in the province and approved by the licensing authorities. The purpose of this requirement is to estimate the applicant's moral, social and ethical characteristics as well as to form an idea of his general and professional education."[16] In addition an immigrant physician is expected to read and write English or French, and in most provinces, he must show that he intends to become a Canadian citizen. But the immigrant physician's trials are not over; he must then obtain an Enabling Certificate which grants him permission to write the examinations of the Medical Council of Canada.

The care which licensing authorities take to ensure that alien physicians reach the educational standards of native-born Canadian physicians, and seemingly the educational standards reached by physicians registered on

14 / Provincial Medical Board of Nova Scotia, *Brief Submitted to the Royal Commission on Health Services*, Halifax: October 1961, p. 8.

15 / S. Judek, *Medical Manpower in Canada*, Royal Commission on Health Services, Ottawa: Queen's Printer, 1964, p. 35.

16 / *Ibid.*

the General List of the Medical Council of Great Britain, might appear to reflect their concern with the maintenance of the standards of practice. But apparently, once the physician is registered to practise, he can continue to do so with only the informal controls of colleagues and the obvious sanctions of the law to ensure that standards are maintained. Once the physician has been licensed the licensing body shows little concern with standards unless colleagues or members of the public present evidence of medical care of poor quality. In other words, despite the claims of licensing authorities concerning standards of competence these evidently require little if any formal professional scrutiny after initial registration to practise, except in the hospital where the Medical Advisory Committee and its various sub-committees may seek to control professional behaviour.

The claim of the licensing bodies is that their concern with the qualifications of alien physicians is based upon their responsibility to see that standards of medical practice are maintained. But regardless of the validity of this claim, it is obvious that by limiting the inflow of alien physicians in this manner the growth in the supply of physicians is restricted and the economic security of the practising profession is more assured.

THE MEDICAL COUNCIL OF CANADA

National uniform minimum qualification standards is the intent of the Canada Medical Act of 1910 which came into force in 1912. This Act was the basis for the establishment of the Medical Council of Canada. The Council consists of:

A   three members appointed by the Governor General in Council;
B   two members representing each province who shall be elected under regulations to be made in that behalf by the provincial medical council;
C   one member from each University or Incorporated Medical School or College in Canada having an arrangement with a University for the conferring of degrees on its graduates;
D   three members who shall be elected by the homeopathic practitioners in Canada, each of whom shall reside in a different province.[17]

In order to maintain uniformly high professional standards throughout Canada the Council conducts examinations of medical students who have fulfilled the other existing requirements for registration with the provincial colleges.

17 / Medical Council of Canada, *Brief Submitted to the Royal Commission on Health Services*, Ottawa: March 1962, p. 2.

Although there may be variations between provinces, the procedures which an aspiring physician must undertake in order to obtain a licence from the provincial College of Physicians and Surgeons are as follows: (*a*) graduate from a recognized university medical school whose curriculum must at least be recognized by the College, (*b*) meet the educational requirements of the College for the granting of an Enabling Certificate which permits the individual to write the Medical Council of Canada examinations, (*c*) complete one year of internship in a Canadian hospital approved by the Canadian Medical Association for junior intern training or in a United States hospital affiliated with a university and approved by the College for this purpose, (*d*) pass the examinations set by the Medical Council of Canada, (*e*) be a Canadian citizen or possess the requisite immigrant status.

It is apparent that the right of Canadian universities with medical schools to confer degrees in medicine is restricted by the right of the Medical Council of Canada, and of the provincial Colleges of Physicians and Surgeons, to control examinations and educational standards. The Medical Council, on which university medical schools are represented but which they do not control, must satisfy itself that the universities' examinations are of a satisfactory standard by prescribing its own examination prior to registration. MacFarlane points out that attempts have been made to have the conferring of the MD degree accepted as qualification for registration.

Periodically suggestions are made that the passing of the final year examinations in Canadian medical schools and the conferring of a degree in medicine should in itself be sufficient evidence on which the Medical Council of Canada could give the student registration.... The question of automatic registration for graduates of Canadian medical schools has been debated on more than one occasion during the last 15 years in the Medical Council of Canada, but the proposal has been defeated.[18]

According to Judek the opposite situation has occurred. "Most of the medical schools have accepted the MCC examinations, in whole or in part, as their own final examinations."[19]

THE ROYAL COLLEGE OF PHYSICIANS AND SURGEONS

The requirements for postgraduate training in medical specialties are set out by the Royal College of Physicians and Surgeons of Canada. The

18 / J. A. MacFarlane, *Medical Education in Canada*, Royal Commission on Health Services, Ottawa: Queen's Printer, 1964, p. 85.
19 / Judek, *Medical Manpower*, p. 33.

business of the College is the responsibility of a Council consisting of the immediate past president and twenty-four fellows elected on a regional basis. It has the power to hold special examinations for physicians seeking specialty status and to determine the nature of these examinations and other qualifications. Fellowship in the College is determined on the basis of the applicant's qualifications as determined by College examination in either a medical or a surgical specialty before a board of examiners appointed by the Council. The medical specialties represented in the College in 1962 were internal medicine, anaesthesia, bacteriology, dermatology, neurology, paediatrics, pathology, physical medicine and rehabilitation, psychiatry, diagnostic radiology, and therapeutic radiology; the surgical specialties were general surgery, cardiovascular and thoracic surgery, neurosurgery, obstetrics and gynaecology, ophthalmology, orthopaedic surgery, otolaryngology, plastic surgery, and urology.[20]

The main function of the College is the control of the development of graduate medical education. It "sets standards of training in the medical and surgical specialties, approves hospitals and institutions in which such training may be taken in Canada, scrutinizes the credentials and qualifications of all those applying to take its examinations and conducts specialist examinations at two levels at somewhat different standards."[21] The standards of training required by the College in the particular specialties are prescribed in detail and cover both the basic science and the clinical requirements for a specialty. Besides meeting these technical requirements the candidate for a fellowship must satisfy the Council that he has graduated from a medical school approved by the College and that he has the requisite moral and ethical standing.[22]

Much of the work of the Council is undertaken by committees of fellows. The Committee on Ethics is the body which ensures that the professional conduct of a fellow conforms with the norms laid down in the uniform code of ethics adopted by the College and other professional organizations in medicine. In fact, before he can be recognized as a fellow of the College, an aspiring candidate must sign a declaration to the effect that his conduct will be guided by the code of ethics and he waives certain rights on being accepted by the College. In the course of his professional career, should he be judged guilty of unethical conduct by the Council his name may be erased from the list of fellows. By signing the declaration he "specifically waives any right or claim to damages in the

20 / Royal College of Physicians and Surgeons of Canada, *Brief Submitted to the Royal Commission on Health Services*, Ottawa: February 1962, pp. 2–3. Much of the discussion concerning the College which follows is based on this source.
21 / *Ibid.*, p. 5.
22 / *Ibid.*, p. 6.

event of his being removed."[23] The code of ethics specifies the normative behaviour expected of the physician in his relations with a patient with regard to a patient's confidences, costs of treatment, professional standards, and the maintenance of standards. It also specifies a number of other responsibilities of the physicians.

A physician attending a patient must endeavour to consult with another physician in cases which are difficult or obscure, but the consultant must report and discuss his findings with the attending physician. The induction or procuring of abortion is "a violation both of the moral law and of the Criminal Code of Canada, except when there is justification for its performance." In the course of friendship with the patient of another physician, the physician must not interfere in the treatment of the attending physician. A physician must endeavour to maintain high quality of service. He should not treat himself or members of his family for serious illness if "the services of another physician are available." He must not attempt to advertise a commodity. He should only charge a fee for "work actually done for the patient," according to fee standards adopted by the profession. He should not advertise in any form: "Practice should not be gathered by any kind of solicitation, direct or indirect. The best advertisement of a physician is a well-merited reputation for ability and probity in his profession." When he communicates opinions on medical subjects to the public they "should be presented as from some organized and recognized medical society or association and not from an individual physician." If he takes part in a discussion on radio the physician "should avoid methods which tend to his personal professional advantage." Should a physician make a scientific discovery it "should be made common for the advantage of the whole profession, and for the progress of science." The ethical responsibilities of the physician are applicable in group or any other type of practice.

A physician called to a case in the absence of the attending physician or in emergency must hand over all responsibility for the case when the attending physician arrives. A physician who has been an assistant to another physician "should not begin practice in the same neighbourhood except with the written consent of the practitioner for whom he has substituted or to whom he has been an assistant." He should obtain the patient's consent by signature before supplying information on forms requiring medical reports by the physician. Contract practice is unethical "if there is solicitation for patients, underbidding, interference with the choice of physician, or if the compensation is so low that adequate service cannot be

23 / Royal College of Physicians and Surgeons of Canada, *Act of Incorporation, Constitution By-Laws, and Code of Ethics,* Ottawa: 1959, p. 14.

given, or if professional services are made to yield profits to controlling lay groups." If physicians cannot settle differences between themselves, "they should be referred to the appropriate authority. Complaints of unprofessional conduct should be referred in writing to the Registrar of the provincial licensing authority." If he should be required to appear in court as a medical witness a physician should try to help the court to arrive at a just decision. He must "not make use of, or recommend any remedy, the principal ingredients of which are not disclosed to the profession." He cannot assume the care "of a patient who has had another attendant in the current illness, unless he has satisfied himself that those responsible have notified the other physician that his services are no longer required." When he takes over the care of a patient from another physician "he should make no adverse comment upon the treatment already given." He may apply for a position on the attending staff of a hospital "but should not canvass for it." In his relations with nurses the physician should "support and where necessary, guide the work of nurses. ..."[24]

As part of its educational role the College has a programme of approval of hospitals in Canada for graduate training in medicine. This is the responsibility of a Committee on Approval of Hospitals for Advanced Graduate Training which has laid down "criteria for the quantitative and qualitative assessment of hospitals applying for approval of resident training programmes."[25] The actual evaluation of specialist training facilities according to these criteria is undertaken by the Canadian Council on Hospital Accreditation at the request of the College. Hospital specialist training programmes accredited in this manner are subject to periodic review.

This Council was set up in 1950 and consists of five representatives from the Canadian Hospital Association, four representatives from the Canadian Medical Association, two representatives from the Royal College of Physicians and Surgeons of Canada, and one representative from l'Association des médecins de langue française du Canada. The Council, as a corporate body, has the right to survey Canadian hospitals and to accredit them on the basis of prescribed standards of hospital organization and administration and patient care. It also has the right "to assist and cooperate with Canadian organizations having programmes of approval of hospitals for medical internship and for advanced graduate medical training."[26]

24 / *Ibid.*, pp. 27–35.
25 / Royal College of Physicians and Surgeons of Canada, *Brief Submitted to the Royal Commission on Health Services*, p. 13.
26 / Canadian Council on Hospital Accreditation, *Brief Submitted to the Royal Commission on Health Services*, Toronto: May 1962, p. 3.

In 1962 about two-thirds of all hospitals approved by the College for graduate training in medical and surgical specialties were affiliated with university medical schools.[27] In recent years a few universities in Canada have commenced the planning or actual building of university hospitals which, like the university-affiliated hospital, will undertake the education of undergraduate students in medicine, and medical interns, as well as graduate training in medicine.

The power of the Royal College of Physicians and Surgeons is obvious. It has the power to recognize specialties; to determine the educational content of graduate specialty training programmes in hospitals and elsewhere; to decide which hospitals shall be accredited for graduate training; to specify the type and content of specialty examinations; to assess the moral and ethical acceptability of candidates for fellowships; and to judge the subsequent professional behaviour of the specialist. It controls not only the educational preparation and subsequent behaviour of the specialist, but through the standards it lays down for specialty training it effectively controls standards in hospitals which it accredits for graduate training.

THE COLLEGE OF GENERAL PRACTICE

In order to prevent the deterioration of their professional status in the eyes of the public, as well as their specialist colleagues, the general practitioners, with the assistance of the Canadian Medical Association, formed the College of General Practice in 1954. Its founders recognized that the prestige of the general practitioner was lower than that of his specialist colleagues and that in order to raise it the general practitioner must compete for status with the specialist. Success in status competition between groups within a profession depends to a large extent on a group's control over its members particularly with regard to training and performance and the acceptance by the profession and the community of the group's claims concerning the uniqueness and superiority of the services its members provide. The function of the College of General Practice is to promote in medical schools the development of curricula suitable for general practice; to develop programmes of postgraduate education, continuing postgraduate education, and in-hospital postgraduate residency training; to promote the integration of the general practitioners into hospital staffs, the recognition of his distinctive services, and the maintenance of the standard of these services.[28] The College has had some success in promoting the development of curricula, and, as indicated previously, it has laid

27 / *Ibid.*, p. 15.
28 / College of General Practice of Canada, *Brief Submitted to the Royal Commission on Health Services*, Toronto: May 1962, pp. 6–7.

down educational requirements for active membership[29] but lacking the statutory authority to control the educational preparation of general practitioners it is doubtful whether these requirements can succeed in raising their standards of competence, and thereby assist them in their competition for status with the specialists.

In its claims concerning the distinctive nature of the services provided by a general practitioner, the College has sought to cast the specialist in an unfavourable light by stressing that increased medical specialization has created an emphasis on organ systems of the body and on episodic illness rather than continuing medical care, and an impersonal attitude towards patient care. But though the College claims that the services provided by the general practitioner are somehow unique and of special value, its specification of this uniqueness and value gives the impression that many of the characteristics it sets forth could be applied equally to the specialist: for example, the general practitioner "does not confine his work to a special field and his services include: (A) Early diagnostic and therapeutic services, (B) General availability, (C) Continuity of service, (D) The promotion of health, (E) The prevention of disease."[30]

There can be little doubt that general practitioners face severe competition for status from specialists and that, in order to maintain some semblance of their former status, they are forced to redefine their professional role. But medical knowledge and technology are the allies of the specialist rather than the general practitioner, with the result that in order to maintain his position the general practitioner must try to compete with the specialist on the latter's terms by seeking control of educational standards and role performance.

Specialists and hospital officials have recognized the difficulties which general practitioners face in trying to maintain acceptable standards of performance. Many hospitals are reluctant to allow some of the practitioners hospital privileges partly for this reason. The difficulties which such a practitioner faces in attempting to carry out his professional role under this handicap are obvious, and it is for these, as well as other reasons, that the College of General Practice has sought to raise the professional standards of general practitioners while attempting to lower the barriers to the granting of hospital privileges to some general practitioners. In its supplementary brief to the Royal Commission on Health Services, the College claimed "that some hospitals practise a form of discrimination against the general practitioners as a group."[31] The College insisted that

---

29 / See p. 50.
30 / College of General Practice of Canada, *Brief*, pp. 9–10.
31 / College of General Practice of Canada, *Supplementary Brief Submitted to the Royal Commission on Health Services*, Toronto: August 1962, p. 1.

this restriction applied not only to some community hospitals but to university teaching hospitals as well, and urged that this barrier be lifted and that the general practitioner should be accepted as an active member of the hospital medical staff and recognized as a physician who could admit patients. This action would require those hospitals accepting these proposals of the College to set up departments of general practice[32] in which general practitioners would have the same hospital privileges as specialists although they would not necessarily have the same level of training and skill. The College has had only partial success in persuading general and teaching hospitals to give general practitioners full admitting privileges and to set up departments of general practice.

The difficulty which the College encounters in its attempts to persuade hospitals to grant the general practitioner admitting privileges and a separate hospital department is due, in large part, to the reluctance of the Canadian Council on Hospital Accreditation to accept the claims of the College concerning the rights and qualifications of the general practitioner. Under its Letters Patent the Council has the statutory powers to specify standards governing hospital accreditation.[33] It specifies that in general hospitals of 75 or more beds, medical staff should be departmentalized in terms of clinical services. The qualifications of departmental personnel, and the qualifications, method of appointment, and functions of the heads of departments are laid down with the exception of a department of general practice which is not a required department of such a hospital. Where a department of general practice is organized the Council specifies that its function "shall be limited to administration and education. It shall not be a clinical service and no patients shall be admitted to the department."[34] The Council further specifies that the general practitioners who are members of a department of general practice must provide their services in other departments, be bound by the rules of these departments, and accept the authority of the heads of these departments.[35]

The Canadian Council on Hospital Accreditation in fact places the general practitioner in a subordinate professional role to the specialist in the hospital, and leaves it to the hospital to decide if a department of general practice should be set up. Since the College does not have a statutory control equivalent to that of the College of Physicians and Surgeons at either the provincial or the federal level, it does not have the power to raise or protect the professional status of the general practitioner.

32 / *Ibid.*, p. 2.
33 / Canadian Council on Hospital Accreditation, *Brief*, Appendix B, pp. 3–4.
34 / *Ibid.*, Appendix D, p. 12.
35 / *Ibid.*

SPECIALTY ORGANIZATIONS

Organizations similar in function to that of the College of General Practice also exist in the area of specialty practice. Each recognized specialty has some form of association whose aim is to promote the interest and maintain the standards of practice of a particular specialty, but like the College they have no statutory disciplinary function. These societies of specialists sometimes disseminate scientific information in the area of specialization which they represent through the publication of journals and by holding periodic meetings of specialists.

THE CANADIAN MEDICAL ASSOCIATION

The organization that seeks to bring together all physicians, both general practitioners and specialists, into a cohesive group with the aim of promoting the interests of all its members is the Canadian Medical Association, with its provincial divisions each of which is autonomous within its particular province. The executive policy-making body of the Association is the General Council comprised of approximately 180 members. The executive committee of the Council includes one representative of each of the provincial divisions as well as officers of the Association.

Membership in the Association is based on membership in the provincial division, which is voluntary in all except three provinces. In Saskatchewan the provincial Association was merged with the provincial College of Physicians and Surgeons. In Alberta, "the compulsory annual licence fee supports both the College and the Association, and in New Brunswick a similar system obtains."[36]

The activities of the Association are carried out by numerous committees of which there are two types, standing and special. National policy regarding specific areas of activity and concern emerge from the deliberations of these committees which are usually composed of the chairmen of the corresponding provincial committees.[37] These committees cover a wide range of activities which Taylor classifies as "(a) medical practices and standards; and (b) the organizing and financing of medical services."[38] The federal nature of the Association, as reflected in the interlocking of provincial interests in committees, assures a high degree of national consensus on the important policy matters. In fact, as one reads the briefs which each of the provincial divisions submitted to the Royal

36 / Taylor, "The Role of the Medical Profession," p. 112.
37 / *Ibid.*
38 / *Ibid.*

Commission on Health Services one is struck by the degree of agreement in these briefs on major matters of interest to the profession. To give one example of the many instances where this occurred: on the subject of health insurance the British Columbia Division of the Canadian Medical Association recommended to the Commission,

That voluntary prepaid health insurance be recognized as the system best suited to the needs of ... British Columbia ... that premiums for those who cannot afford them be paid from public funds, and be paid as premiums to one or more of the existing voluntary plans ... and that the number and variety of voluntary plans operating in B.C. be encouraged both as a competitive control measure and as a means of making differing degrees and types of insurance available to all.[39]

On the same topic, the Canadian Medical Association recommended to the Commission,

That, for the 1,520,000 persons, or approximately 8% of Canada's population who may be adjudged to be medically indigent, tax funds be used to provide comprehensive medical insurance on a service basis ... That approved carriers of medical services insurance be selected from the plans now operating under voluntary auspices or from plans now providing social assistance medical services to provide insurance coverage for those persons aided from public funds.[40]

The similarity in the intent of both these statements is obvious. A similar consensus could be indicated for every other major area of interest.

These interests are promoted in a number of ways, of which Taylor describes four.[41] The most obvious of these is through the press, a course open to any other interest group, and through personal contact which, in the case of the physician, is a personal contact of a special kind. The second promotional channel is the formal or informal contacts between the profession and the government. Many senior officials of government health departments are physicians, including sometimes the provincial minister of health. "In one western province the Deputy Minister of Health served five years simultaneously as Secretary of the Medical Association. In some other provinces the minister or deputy minister is a member *ex officio* of the executive of the provincial division." Having undertaken the same type of training and education as their colleagues in the community they will share common values and perspectives. The

39 / Canadian Medical Association, BC Division, *Brief Submitted to the Royal Commission on Health Services*, Vancouver: February 1962, p. S5.

40 / Canadian Medical Association, *Brief Submitted to the Royal Commission on Health Services*, Toronto: May 1962, pp. 7–8.

41 / Taylor, "The Role of the Medical Profession." Taylor's description, which follows, can be consulted in pages 115–18 of his article.

General Council of the Canadian Medical Association includes representatives of various departments of the federal government including the Deputy Minister of Health.

Another means by which professional interests are promoted is through what Taylor terms "institutional patterns." By this he means arrangements such as the medical care prepayment plans in the area of health insurance. "They are large, successfully operating agencies, cast in such a mould as to institutionalize the profession's principles and practices, and these are further strengthened by the contractual relations into which these agencies enter through collective bargaining agreements between management and labour."

The last type of arrangement mentioned by Taylor through which the profession's interests are promoted is termed the "tie-in-endorsement" in which the medical profession is "tied-in" with other groups such as the other health professions, hospital associations, and the insurance industry seeking to protect similar interests and policies.

The strength of these influences depends on the degree of cohesion of the Association. This is generated through the cross-membership in the committees of the Association at both federal and provincial levels and through the type and degree of control exerted in the provincial division. For example, in Saskatchewan and Alberta the licensing and disciplinary powers and the promotion of professional interests – the political function – are the responsibility of the same body, the provincial division. The extent to which the pursuit of the political aims of the association can be facilitated through the threat of licensing and disciplinary sanctions where the political, licensing, and disciplinary functions are the functions of one body is evident in the dispute in Saskatchewan between the provincial government and the College of Physicians and Surgeons of that province concerning the introduction of the Saskatchewan Medical Care Insurance Act of 1961,[42] and in its aftermath which resulted in the emergence of community clinics. The clinics were organized by group practices to serve the health needs of communities and staffed by physicians, some of whom were recent immigrants, who supported the Medical Care Insurance Act to which the majority of their professional colleagues were opposed. Although the clinic physicians were licensed by the Saskatchewan College of Physicians and Surgeons they claimed that they had been prevented from gaining admitting privileges in a number of hospitals in the province. "Admitting privileges are granted formally by hospital boards but since these boards are composed of lay persons they must depend on committees of staff doctors for advice with respect to the granting of admitting

42 / E. A. Tollefson, *Bitter Medicine*, Saskatoon: Modern Press, 1963.

privileges. And a considerable number of clinic doctors claim that those committees of hospital doctors have discriminated against them in the advice which they have given to the hospital boards."[43] The government appointed a royal commission to investigate these complaints and it found that in each case the problem was "attributable to the marked division of opinion among Saskatchewan physicians as to how medicine should be practiced."[44] The Report of the Commission "appears to leave little doubt that the withholding of hospital privileges is being used by the organized medical profession as a weapon in its fight with community clinics and their doctors."[45]

The dispute between the Saskatchewan government and the medical profession in that province strengthened the bonds between members of the latter group. In this type of cohesive in-group physicians deal with each other on a personal level, and are united in the face of outside criticism and hostility which in many cases are based upon the outsider's concern with what he sees as a gap between the universalistic service goals of the medical profession and the actual behaviour of its individual members.

It is this constant striving to rationalize universal goals and self-interest, particularly in an era of rapid social change when the status, standards of service, and economic security of the profession are threatened that the physician finds most difficult. Caught in the press of change he is subtly coerced through informal professional controls to maintain practices which, while serving professional self-interests, widen the gap between his actions and these goals. The role strains which result are probably the most severe of any professional role, and, as the Saskatchewan experience indicates, sometimes result in a breakdown of informal group controls. As these controls weaken, internal dissension grows and becomes obvious to the consumer of the group's services. In this way, outsiders become involved in the issues between the opposing factions in the professional group. Group cohesion can be reintroduced by the imposition of stronger controls, both formal and informal, but unless these controls are changed to meet changing conditions within medicine, such as the growth of medical knowledge and technology, and outside medicine, such as the increasing role of government in meeting consumer demands and the rising expectations of the consumers themselves, the gap between the universalistic goals of the profession and the behaviour demanded of the physician in pursuit of his self-interest increases.

43 / W. P. Thompson, *Medical Care*, Toronto: Clarke, Irwin & Co. Ltd., 1964, p. 87.
44 / The Honourable Justice Mervyn Woods, *Report on Hospital Staff Appointments*, Regina: 1963, p. 99.
45 / Thompson, *Medical Care*, p. 88.

The foregoing analysis of the structure and functions of both voluntary and non-voluntary professional associations has shown that the manner in which the power of the licensing authority has been used has had functional consequences for medical education and medical practice. The state has delegated the licensing power to the profession, which has used it to create standards of entry and to enforce a mode of professional behaviour upon its members. While leaving the medical school its traditional function of educating the student physician, the profession has used its power to stipulate the type of medical education to be given by the medical school and the values to be instilled into medical students in this process. This control has given the profession a supply of new members who, having undergone the socializing process of the medical school, are a more or less uniform product in terms of technical training and social attitudes. In the remaining years of technical training the profession uses its licensing power to lay down further technical requirements and modes of professional behaviour. The consequence of this second stage for the aspiring physician is that he becomes an even more uniform product showing skills, attitudes, and social perspectives which generate a resistance to change in medical education, the organization of medical practice, and professional licensing and control.

The extent to which other professional bodies control the educational process of their student practitioners is difficult to assess. Comparative sociological studies of this nature analysing the way in which professional control of licensing results in professional control of other features of professional life are scarce, but recent developments in Ontario universities in the appraisal of postgraduate programmes offer some evidence that the control of professional education in the sciences, social sciences, and humanities can be retained by the university with no deterioration of professional quality standards. The university, even though responsible for the technical education of a range of professions, is in a position through its academic senate to assure that the highest possible educational standards are maintained for each. In maintaining such standards it does not need to be influenced by the pressures or ditcates of a professional licensing body. Now that universities are being asked to undertake the additional responsibility for programmes of continuing medical education which will assist in maintaining these standards throughout the professional life of the practitioner, it may not appear unreasonable for them to suggest that they have some responsibility in certain aspects of the licensing function.

7

THE DEVELOPMENT OF
MEDICAL CARE
INSURANCE PROGRAMMES

MANY PHYSICIANS claim that the doctor-patient relationship must remain untouched by the intervention of third parties. The claim ignores the fact that such intervention has occurred throughout history. The code of Hammurabi, nearly 4,300 years old, specified the penalties which a third party may impose should a physician fail to meet public expectations. "If a doctor shall treat a gentleman and shall open an abscess with a bronze knife and shall preserve the eye of the patient, he shall receive ten shekels of silver.... If the doctor shall open an abscess with a bronze knife and shall kill the patient or shall destroy the sight of the eye, his hands shall be cut off."[1] Present-day third party sanctions are not so obviously coercive, but their existence is evident, for example in newspaper accounts of malpractice suits against practising physicians and in the legal requirements that physicians must divulge before a court of law "the contents of this 'privileged' relationship if failure to do so results in endangering the public welfare or would unwarrantedly prejudice the outcome of a legal action."[2]

Another form of third party intervention, one that today appears to many physicians of paramount importance to their conditions of work, comprises those institutional arrangements that have emerged to finance the cost of medical care. These arrangements are based on a polarity of opposing values: those founded on voluntary participation as against those created by compulsory participation. The voluntary arrangements include the indemnity contracts sold by commercial insurance companies, the service contracts of the prepayment plans sponsored by the medical profession, and the plans organized by co-operatives and fraternal organizations for their members which follow general insurance principles. The

1 / As quoted in Herman M. Somers and Anne R. Somers, *Doctors, Patients, and Health Insurance*, Washington: The Brookings Institution, 1961, pp. 218–19.
2 / *Ibid.*, p. 220.

compulsory arrangements include those administered by governments and organized on a universal, comprehensive basis. A significant development in the organizational pattern of medical care insurance is the emergence of plans which are based on voluntary participation but which are administered by a government agency responsible for enrolment, the collection of premiums, and the payment of fees to physicians for services rendered under the plan. By July 1, 1967, three such plans were in operation: the Ontario Medical Services Insurance Plan, the British Columbia Insurance Plan, and the Alberta Health Plan. The development of these three plans will be discussed in the following chapter.

The nature and development of a particular professional ideology can be studied by analysing that profession's reactions to the changing conditions of work. In the case of the medical profession in Canada the reaction that is most significant in this connection is the one to medical care insurance, and the nature of this reaction is determined by the profession's perception of the extent to which this type of third party intervention can affect working conditions. The profession realizes that the power of the state to control the conditions of work far exceeds that of any other type of third party. Thus the prospect of government control of certain conditions of practice, particularly the amount and type of remuneration, generates strain and anxiety on the part of the physician, but voluntary medical care insurance and prepayment, although the type of third party arrangement preferred by the profession, creates similar strains and anxieties. Thus all the institutional mechanisms which have emerged to finance the cost of medical care, voluntary or government, have their attendant strains. The profession seeks to protect its interests, as we shall show later, by stressing and reiterating basic ideological beliefs and values, some of which are linked to society-wide beliefs and values and others are distinctive to the profession. In order to understand the medical profession's ideological reaction to government medical care insurance in particular, some analysis of the organization, development, and consequences for the physician's role of voluntary medical care insurance is particularly important since these factors appear so frequently in ideological statements of the profession.

VOLUNTARY MEDICAL CARE INSURANCE

The two basic types of voluntary medical care insurance can be distinguished according to the parties to the contract. The commercial insurance company contracts with an individual to reimburse him for some proportion of the medical expenses he has acquired as a result of illness.

The prepayment plan does not contract with the individual to provide for this indemnification. Instead, it arranges with the physicians agreeing to participate in the scheme to pay them directly for the whole or part of the cost of the medical care they have provided to individual subscribers to the scheme. Berry makes the distinction between the two types of contract in the following terms:

The essential distinction lies in the carrier's obligation. The insurance carrier accepts an obligation to make cash payments to the subscriber in the event of certain occurrences. The prepayment carrier ... accepts responsibility for the compensation of a participating physician who renders necessary medical care or services. This latter is the basis for the term "service contract" as opposed to "indemnity contract" – the subscriber receives *services* not cash payments.[3]

The insurance contract attempts to protect the insured against the loss of income due to the cost of medical care by paying him all or part of the medical expenses incurred during illness. The prepayment contract attempts to provide medical care for those requiring it by paying the physician, on a fee-for-service basis, not the recipient of services. Prepayment systems of medical care not only attempt to lessen the risk of high medical expenses, but also to provide for a more adequate distribution of medical services without placing restrictions on the physicians' earning power. As these two types of contracts have developed they have affected each other to the extent that today each includes certain elements of the other.

There are five types of voluntary medical care insurance carriers: stock insurance companies and mutual insurance companies, both of which are commercial carriers; the prepayment plans which are physician-sponsored and oriented towards the provision of services; the co-operative and fraternal plans which, although primarily commercially oriented, possess a degree of service orientation; and the government-administered plans in Ontario, British Columbia and Alberta. The benefits offered by the various plans can vary widely, ranging from surgical procedures or medical care only to comprehensive benefits which include most, if not all, the medical procedures and care required during an illness.

Recent data published by the federal Department of National Health and Welfare indicate the population covered by both government and voluntary medical care insurance plans at the end of 1966. At that time over 16 million Canadians, or 82 per cent of the population, had some

3 / Charles H. Berry, *Voluntary Medical Insurance and Prepayment*, Royal Commission on Health Services, Ottawa: Queen's Printer, 1964, p. 4. The discussion of the structure and function of insurance and prepayment schemes which follows is based on this source.

form of insurance to meet the cost of medical care. Of this percentage, 67.7 per cent were enrolled in voluntary plans, and 13.9 per cent in government plans.[4] This 1966 figure of 82 per cent is a substantial increase over the 59 per cent estimated by the Royal Commission on Health Services five years earlier.[5]

The Royal Commission on Health Services had some interesting comments to make regarding the cost of voluntary medical care insurance and the retention costs involved in operating the plans:

In 1961, the insurance and prepayment systems paid on behalf of 9.6 million Canadians, medical bills, and in some cases some related other bills, totalling $175,122,600, an average of $18.20 per person. For this purpose and for the advantages of insurance, these 9.6 million Canadians paid in premiums $224,093,200 or an average of $23.28 per person. The retention figure – i.e., the costs of administration, acquisition of new groups or individuals, commissions, taxes, and profits, – totalled $49 million, or an extra 28 percent added to the amount of the payments for medical services.

The retention figure is highest among the commercial companies, reaching 38 percent for group contracts, but rising to 151 percent for non-group contracts sold to individual purchasers. This latter figure means that for each dollar of protection, the individual would have paid $2.51 in premiums. By contrast, the prepayment plans actually paid a higher proportion of premiums for medical services on behalf of non-group subscribers than of group subscribers, with retention figures of 11 percent and 18 percent, respectively. The retention figures for commercial carriers covering group and group contracts was 44.3 percent and the corresponding figure for prepayment plans was 17.6 percent.[6]

This system of insurance and prepayment coverage has a variety of consequences for a number of social groups. There can be little doubt that it has alleviated the risk of the heavy and sometimes catastrophic cost of illness for the patient and provided greater economic security for the physician in the sense that he now receives payment for some services which traditionally he has provided free. On the other hand, the system leaves significant numbers of people uncovered and therefore exposed to the risks of the cost of illness and it carries a heavy "overhead" cost, particularly in the case of the commercial insurance companies.

Of major importance for this analysis are the consequences of this "third party" system for the role of the physician. The physician-sponsored

4 / Canada, Department of National Health and Welfare, *Provincial Health Services by Program*, Ottawa: 1968, p. 167.
5 / Royal Commission on Health Services, *Final Report*, vol. I, p. 727.
6 / *Ibid.*, p. 732.

prepayment schemes are particularly important in this regard. The increasing involvement of physicians in these organizations coincides with the increasing demand for universal health insurance since World War II. In order to meet the demands of consumers of medical care for some alleviation of the financial hazards of illness physicians have sponsored, and sometimes actively engaged in, the organization of voluntary prepayment medical care schemes.

Physicians sponsoring prepayment schemes saw them as a mechanism which would provide medical care insurance on their terms rather than those of the government. This view is evident in briefs presented to the Royal Commission on Health Services by the Canadian Medical Association and physician-sponsored prepayment plans. The Canadian Medical Association indicated that it wished to maintain the measure of authority the medical profession and its members enjoy under the existing medical care plans. In the brief of Trans-Canada Medical Plans the claim is made that among its member plans there are varying degrees of public administrative representation, but it is the medical profession which applies quality controls on participating physicians. These physician-sponsored plans have not attempted to control the quality of medical care, but have provided a vehicle for the profession to exercise this responsibility. Nevertheless, the brief argued that the method of operation of these plans had led to better quality of medical care through scrutiny of the physician's patterns of practice. This organization also claimed that the physician's authority would be undermined if control of the physician-sponsored plans were to be taken from the profession and given to government or another third party.[7]

Various control mechanisms are becoming an accepted element in physician-sponsored prepayment plans despite the physicians' desire to retain control over the conditions of practice. These mechanisms are directed at maintaining financial stability by curbing demands on the part of subscribers for unnecessary services and restricting physicians seeking to provide these services. According to a spokesman for Trans-Canada Medical Plans these various control arrangements have been accepted by participating physicians.

Each plan maintains an individual record of each covered subscriber and of each physician; this offers many advantages for medical assessors and medical committees in carrying out their duties. For unusual claims and those of a problem nature medical reference committees or other similar types of arrangements are available, through the facilities of the provincial medical

7 / Trans-Canada Medical Plans, *Brief Submitted to the Royal Commission on Health Services*, Toronto: May 1962.

division, for assistance in adjudication. This reservoir of knowledge and experience provides tremendous assistance to the plan administration in carrying out this phase of its responsibility. As a means of assisting in a high level of medical and economic soundness, the providers of care have ... participated ... in the creation and maintainance of various control arrangements developed in cooperation with their member plans.[8]

The practising physician who is a participating member of a physician-sponsored prepayment plan faces severe cross pressures. Knowing that his claims for services rendered to patients may be reviewed by medical colleagues, he will seek to keep his fees within limits acceptable to the prepayment plan, try to follow acceptable therapeutic procedures, and treat only as many patients as is consistent with acceptable standards of medical care. However, these third party arrangements have increased the number of persons seeking medical services, and since the supply of physicians cannot be expanded quickly to meet increased demand, the individual physician must take on a large case load. Part of his incentive for doing so is that since his fees for this larger patient load will be paid by a third party, and since he will not have to provide any free service to this population, his income will rise. On the other hand he realizes that in meeting these demands for service he must maintain the medical standards demanded by his professional peers whether they be in medical schools, hospitals, in community practice, or officials of prepayment plans. In the event that prepayment plans were to provide medical services on a universal basis the severity of these cross-pressures would be substantially increased unless the supply of physicians was raised to meet the growth in the volume of the demand for medical services attendant upon universal coverage.

Government-sponsored universal medical care insurance creates similar role strains for the physician. There is one important difference however. Physician-sponsored prepayment schemes are usually physician-controlled, but the control in the government-administered universal medical care insurance lies with the legislature, and with the government administrative agency.

THE DEVELOPMENT OF
GOVERNMENT MEDICAL CARE INSURANCE

The prepayment of physicians' fees, as well as other health services, has become an important element in the health policies of successive Canadian governments, both federal and provincial. The demand for the payment

8 / *Ibid.*, p. 28.

of health services from the public purse followed the emergence accompanying industrialization of major health hazards to whole communities and population groups over which the individual had no control. The epidemics of communicable diseases, for example, required such measures as community control of sanitation, public immunization programmes, control of water supplies, and pasteurization of milk. These measures provided ample evidence of the success of community-wide, publicly controlled programmes. They were public health measures organized by government for whole populations. Other health problems were considered the responsibility of the individual.

As public responsibilities in the health field have grown, the demand for some form of publicly administered medical care prepayment has increased. The beginning of this demand can be seen in the action of the British Columbia legislature which in 1919 appointed a Royal Commission to investigate the matter of health insurance. Its report did not result in health insurance legislation. In 1929 another Royal Commission was appointed which reported in 1932. On the basis of its recommendation for the introduction of a partly compulsory and partly voluntary health insurance scheme legislation was drafted and passed but opposition to it became so vociferous that it was not put into effect.[9]

The Alberta Legislature has had a number of inquiries dealing with health insurance. The 1928 inquiry reported in 1929, and was followed in 1932 by another inquiry which reported in 1934. In 1935 a bill to introduce comprehensive health insurance was passed by the legislature, but it was not introduced. According to the Royal Commission on Health Services, "Alberta has had four medical care insurance acts placed upon its statutes. One of these was passed in 1935, but not proclaimed. The second was passed in 1942 and the third in 1946. The 1946 Act did not come into effect and the 1942 Act was repealed in 1953. The present Act was proclaimed in 1963."[10]

The payment of physicians' services by government began in 1916 when the Saskatchewan legislature amended the Rural Municipality Act to allow rural municipal councils to collect taxes to be used to pay physicians a retainer fee. The services paid for in this manner included minor surgery, maternity care, and public health which included the inspection and immunization of school children. During the next twenty-three years

9 / The discussion of the historical development of health insurance in British Columbia and other provinces is based on Royal Commission on Health Services, *Final Report*, vol. I, pp. 383–422. For a discussion of more recent developments see Chapter 8.

10 / *Ibid.*, p. 396.

the Saskatchewan legislation underwent a number of amendments. In 1939, the passage of the Municipal and Medical Hospital Services Act enabled municipalities to levy taxes of up to $50 per family to provide for medical or hospital services. In 1942, a Select Special Committee on Social Security and Health Services was established. Its report recommended that a Commission be set up "to introduce a health insurance programme as proposed by the federal government."[11] Although an Act incorporating this recommendation was passed by the legislature it was not proclaimed. Instead it was replaced by a Health Services Act in 1945 "which provided for a comprehensive range of health services for recipients of public assistance."[12]

In Manitoba the first indication of legislative interest occurred in 1931 when a legislative committee was set up to examine the problem of health insurance. Its report was presented in 1932, but no legislation resulted. In 1945 the legislature enacted the Health Services Act which, among other things, provided for prepaid general practitioners' services. This type of municipal doctor system was subsequently implemented on a limited scale in Alberta and Manitoba.

A significant aspect of this development at the provincial level is its geographic pattern. With the possible exception of Newfoundland, government interest in the problem of health insurance emerged at a later date in the eastern than in the western provinces. For the first fifty-five years of this century legislative interest in government health insurance in the Province of Ontario is almost negligible compared with that in the three westernmost provinces, although in 1935 the government introduced a programme which provided for physicians' services to public assistance recipients. In the province of Quebec and in the Maritime provinces government interest also remained negligible long after the western provinces had shown an active interest in this problem. In 1942 a Commission was appointed in Quebec which in 1943 recommended universal health insurance but no legislative enactment of the proposal followed. In the Maritime provinces no government action in the area of health insurance was evident until recently. In Newfoundland the Cottage Hospital and Medical Care Plan was instituted in 1935. In 1957 a plan was introduced which provided hospital care for children under 16; in 1958 it was expanded to include medical care in hospitals as well.

The reliance on government action in this field in the West was the result of two features of that part of Canada. "In comparison with the

11 / *Ibid.*
12 / *Ibid.*

East, the West suffered two disadvantages; the absence of large fortunes ruled out philanthropy as an adequate means of obtaining needed facilities or for meeting hospital deficits, and sparse settlement made government the most efficacious machinery for solving such problems."[13] However, beyond the regional reference, reliance on government as a major force in the direction of human affairs has been a tradition in Canadian society which grew out of the desire to build a nation largely to counter the threat of American domination. It was this tradition on which the inhabitants of the western provinces of Canada depended when faced with the problem of the provision of health services.

The interest of the federal government in health insurance was first evident in 1928 when the Standing Committee on Industrial and International Relations was given the authority to investigate the problem of insurance against unemployment, sickness, and disability. In 1935 the Employment and Social Insurance Act was passed by the House of Commons, but this Act was ruled unconstitutional by the Supreme Court of Canada and the Privy Council in 1937. In 1939 the Royal Commission on Dominion-Provincial Relations, while recommending that the provinces should accept responsibility for policy regarding the manner in which medical services should be provided for low income groups, suggested "that the Dominion might be in a better position to collect fees for health insurance, especially if there should be a Dominion scheme of compulsory unemployment insurance or contributory old-age pensions."[14] During World War II the problem of health insurance was studied by an advisory committee to the Director of Public Health Services in the Department of Pensions and National Health, and subsequently by the Advisory Committee on Health Insurance. The latter committee submitted its report to a Select Committee on Social Security in 1943. The report was then studied and discussed by the House of Commons Special Committee on Social Security and by witnesses before the Committee. Further hearings were held in 1944 at which time the views of the provinces were elicited at a conference of dominion and provincial ministers and deputy ministers of health. Subsequently, in that year, in its report to the House of Commons the Committee presented a recommended model bill concerning a national health insurance programme.

In August 1945 the federal government called a dominion-provincial Conference on Reconstruction to which it presented a number of objectives for continued economic expansion.[15] According to the federal gov-

---

13 / *Ibid.*, p. 383.   14 / As quoted *ibid.*, p. 400.
15 / Dominion-Provincial Conference on Reconstruction, 1945, *Proposals of the Government of Canada*, p. 7.

ernment, programmes were needed which would expand productive wealth:

The problem is one of devising a sound and consistent programme of public improvements which will expand the productive wealth of the community and widen the opportunities for enterprise and employment. Also we must seek to manage the expenditures on such a programme so that they do not compete with private activity but will supplement it and contribute to the stabilization of employment whenever private employment declines.

The objectives presented to the Conference by the federal government were "high and stable employment and income, and a greater sense of public responsibility for individual economic security and welfare." Among the means for attaining these objectives was the suggestion "to provide, on the basis of small regular payments against large and uncertain individual risks, for such hazards and disabilities as unemployment, sickness and old age."

This Conference, which met both in 1945 and in 1946, became entangled in discussions concerning dominion-provincial financial arrangements, and the federal government's proposals were not accepted. It was not until 1948 with its National Health Grants programme that the federal government became extensively involved in the health services field with the introduction of a scheme to aid the provinces in the strengthening and expansion of their existing health programmes. The grants under this programme were conditional grants-in-aid by the federal government to the provincial government for the development of services related to mental health, tuberculosis control, cancer control, medical rehabilitation and crippled children, child and maternal health; for the stimulation of public health activities and research related to public health; for the training of professional health workers; and for the provision of health facilities.

The prepayment of medical services has been the main focus of the preceding description, but another major element in any public health insurance programme is hospital care. Here, also, it was the western provinces which first introduced government-sponsored hospital care programmes. The first limited programme of this nature was that introduced in Alberta in 1944 which provided for a maximum of twelve days of hospital care for all expectant mothers and their new-born babies. Another limited programme was introduced in Saskatchewan in 1945 which provided hospital care to "all persons in receipt of old age pensions, mothers' allowances, and general relief."[16] This was followed in 1947 by the Saskatchewan Hospital Services Plan. In 1948 the British Columbia Hospital

16 / Royal Commission on Health Services, *Final Report*, vol. I, p. 406.

Insurance Service was introduced and in the following year the Alberta Hospital Services Plan was launched. In 1949 Newfoundland joined the Canadian Confederation and brought with it a limited hospital services plan.[17]

The success of the existing provincial hospital insurance programmes, especially those of Saskatchewan and British Columbia, created an increased demand for similar hospital programmes in those provinces which lacked these health benefits. With the reduction of the shortage of hospital beds and skilled personnel as a result of the National Health Grants programme, a national hospital insurance scheme appeared feasible. In 1955 the federal government called a federal-provincial conference at which the question of a universal comprehensive programme was studied, and by the end of 1956 the essential details of the Hospital Insurance and Diagnostic Services Act had been settled.

Two features of these developments in the introduction of medical care prepayment and hospital insurance, the two major components of a health insurance programme, are significant in the changing public ideology of health insurance. First, compared with the eastern provinces, the western provinces had demographic and economic conditions which were severe obstacles to the provision of an adequate level of health services by the individual, and there was an early acceptance of government action in the provision of these services. Second, although a belief continues to exist among Canadians in *laissez-faire* individualism, especially in economic matters, there is an increasing acceptance at the federal level of government intervention in problems affecting the whole society; in the area of health services such an intervention would take the form of the prepayment of services on a universal basis.

A universal service is one of four different types of provision existing in the contemporary world: "(1) free enterprise; (2) social insurance; (3) public assistance; (4) universal service."[18] The free enterprise pattern is most clearly seen in the United States where the individual is generally responsible for financing his health care. Although a variety of voluntary and public schemes exist to prepay the costs of medical and hospital care, it is the individual's responsibility to seek out appropriate prepayment arrangements. According to one authority, "the growth of health insurance enrollment is inevitably slowing down. It now appears that hospital coverage may taper off at about 75 percent of the civilian population." But, as

17 / *Ibid.*, p. 410.
18 / Milton I. Roemer, "Health Departments and Medical Care: A World Scanning," *Medical Care in Transition*, vol. II, Washington: US Department of Health, Education, and Welfare, 1964, p. 138.

this authority points out, "in view of the modern role of medical care, its costs, and our knowledge of what can be done with insurance, an adequate policy goal requires health insurance protection – private, public, or a mixture of both – for somewhere around 90–95 percent of the people."[19]

In the western continental European countries including France, Germany, the Benelux countries, Italy, Sweden, Norway, and Denmark the social insurance pattern prevails. In these countries medical and hospital services for the most part are provided under social insurance systems. "On the whole ... physicians remain in private medical practice for ambulatory care and receive payments of fees directly or indirectly from the insurance funds."[20]

The public assistance pattern is found mainly in "Asia, Africa, and most of Latin-America, areas characterized as the economically underdeveloped parts of the world. Here the great majority of the population cannot afford to finance needed medical services either through insurance or private payments. They depend for the most part on services provided free by the government and financed from general revenues."[21]

In the western world, Great Britain's National Health Service is the major example of the universal pattern in which contributions are made for health services although the major source of funds to support the operations of the service is general revenues.[22]

There has been a significant stimulus to public acceptance in Canada of the increased role of federal and provincial governments in the prepayment of health services. An important factor was the implementation and public acceptance of the Hospital Insurance programme in the provinces, referred to above, which made hospital services available to all. Another has been the apparent failure of the free enterprise pattern to provide other forms of adequate health care. Two developments are of particular significance in the public acceptance of the increased role of government and the implementation of the universal service pattern of health care: the introduction of medical care insurance in Saskatchewan and the Report of the Royal Commission on Health Services. These are discussed in the next chapter.

19 / Somers and Somers, *Doctors, Patients, and Health Insurance*, pp. 370–71.
20 / Roemer, "Health Departments and Medical Care," p. 139.
21 / *Ibid.*, p. 140.
22 / *Ibid.*, p. 141.

8

GOVERNMENT
MEDICAL CARE INSURANCE

THE INTRODUCTION of government-administered medical care insurance in Saskatchewan on July 1, 1962, was the culmination of a series of developments during the preceding four decades. In 1921 the rural municipalities of Saskatchewan were so sparsely settled that they held little attraction for the physician wishing to practise. The population of these municipalities, however, required medical services. As indicated in the previous chapter, a solution to this problem was the introduction of the initial legislation which allowed the organization of municipal doctor plans through which local residents were taxed to provide sufficient funds to pay the salary of a physician, and the introduction of late-legislation which allowed the municipalities to levy taxes to pay for a wider range of health services including hospital care. This type of prepayment system met the basic needs of the population of rural areas for medical care, and acted as an incentive to physicians to settle in these areas in which, under the traditional organization of private solo practice, they would have found it difficult, if not impossible, to maintain an acceptable income.

Despite the growth of these municipal doctor plans the pressure for a province-wide publicly supported medical care insurance plan increased. In 1942, for example, the Saskatchewan Medical Association stated that it favoured a state-supported health insurance scheme on a fee-for-service basis. In 1944 and 1945 the government and representatives of the Saskatchewan College of Physicians and Surgeons were discussing the feasibility and details of a government medical care programme. The agreement between the government and the profession in Saskatchewan at that time was a reflection of the support for a government health insurance programme by the Canadian Medical Association. The extent of this agreement is evident in the following letter from Premier Douglas of Saskatchewan to Dr. J. L. Brown of the Saskatchewan College of Physicians and Surgeons in September 1945:

September 19, 1945

DEAR DR. BROWN:

I should like first of all to express my appreciation of the opportunities that we have had during the past few months of having frank and open discussions for the purpose of exchanging opinions regarding the problems of administration involved in a Provincial Health Insurance Scheme.

Judging from the slow progress that is being made in the Dominion-Provincial discussions, I expect that it will undoubtedly be a year or two before any health insurance plan is adopted in Saskatchewan. I would therefore like to stress that a final decision in this matter need not be taken immediately. The problem is a serious one and merits continuing discussion between the Government on the one hand and those giving the services on the other. It would therefore appear to me as essential that further discussions would be of mutual benefit and that no hasty decision need be taken in this matter. I would like to suggest further that a negotiating committee be appointed by the College of Physicians and Surgeons with power to act on its behalf.

That being so, and in the light of the discussions we have had, particularly the excellent exchange of opinions which took place last evening, it would seem to me that the following general principles have been agreed upon:

1 That a health insurance scheme in the Province of Saskatchewan shall be administered by a Commission which shall be free from political interference and influence.

2 That this Commission shall be representative of the public (those receiving the service), those giving the service (the various professions concerned), and the Government.

3 The Commission shall have sufficient power and jurisdiction to enable it to establish and to administer a plan which will provide the best possible health insurance plan for the people of this province.

4 The members of the Commission shall be appointed by the Lieutenant-Governor-in-Council and shall consist of:

A   A chairman, who shall be a physician, legally qualified, duly licensed and in good standing in the province, who has had administrative and practical experience in medicine.

B   Representatives of the government, the general public and the following professions:
1 Medicine
2 Dentistry
3 Nursing
4 Pharmacy

It is understood that hospitals will also be represented.

5 No Commissioner, representing a profession, shall be appointed, except with the approval of the profession concerned.

6 The powers of the Commission.

The powers of the Commission shall be as follows:

A The Commission shall have all powers necessary to carry out the objects of the Act and administer the health insurance plan for Saskatchewan.

B While the government is responsible for placing policy before the Commission and for matters of finance, collections, disbursements, audit and reports, the Commission shall nevertheless be independent in the manner and detail of the mechanics necessary to carry this policy into effect and to obtain the objectives desired by the Act.

C The Commission shall have power to return to the government for reconsideration any matters of policy that have been referred to it by the government.

D The professional committees shall have unrestricted jurisdiction over all scientific, technical and professional matters pertaining to their own professions, and the Commission shall be guided by their advice.

E It shall have control of administrative and clerical personnel with powers to hire and discharge subject to the provisions of the Public Service Act.

F In the matter of hiring professional, technical or scientific personnel, the Commission shall consult with the profession concerned regarding the character and standing of the individual in question.

G It shall have the power, subject to the approval of the Minister of Public Health, to make regulations as are necessary to give effect to the health insurance plan.

7 The Commission shall meet at the call of the Chairman whenever necessary but in any event shall meet every three months and shall be called by the Chairman at any time upon written request of three members.

8 The Commission shall establish and appoint from its members a full-time executive committee of three whose chairman shall be the Chairman of the Commission.

9 In addition to the Commission and its executive there shall be advisory committees representing each of the professions providing services, the members of which shall be appointed by the Commission and only with the approval of the professional body concerned. The Commission shall refer to these advisory committees all questions involving professional, technical, and scientific matters and their advice in such matters shall be accepted.

10 Insofar as the medical profession is concerned, the Commission shall refer to the medical advisory committee the following matters, and take action thereon as the medical advisory committee recommends:

A Classification and preparation of lists of physicians, the actual classification of individual physicians to be done by the College of Physicians and Surgeons.

B The general character of the agreement and arrangements where-under the profession will provide medical services.

C All matters regarding authorization and supervision of procedures and treatment.

D The taxing of medical accounts and the adjustments of medical services.
E Regulations to control injustices and abuse of services.
F Determination of what records are confidential and not available for public information or use.
G All other matters of a purely medical nature.

11 Negotiations regarding the rights and conditions of practice of and for physicians under the health insurance scheme shall be conducted between the Commission and the body which is representative of organized medicine in the province, that is, the College of Physicians and Surgeons.

May I suggest again, that you seriously consider the appointment of a negotiating committee representative of the whole medical profession, and invested with full powers to act in its behalf, in order that we may arrive at a mutually satisfactory agreement regarding these matters.

Yours sincerely,
T. C. Douglas.[1]

Three important developments in the eventual introduction of medical care insurance in the province were the election of a government dedicated to collectivist principles, the introduction of hospital insurance, and the growth of government tax-supported and voluntary prepayment medical care plans. In Saskatchewan the collectivist emphasis on medical care emerged clearly with the election of the Co-operative Commonwealth Federation as the government of the province in 1944. The CCF party had fought an election campaign with a political platform which included a promise of health insurance. The medical profession was now faced with the possibility of legislation which appeared to contradict the fundamental beliefs of many physicians concerning the nature of medicine and the organization of medical practice. The promised legislation was based on the belief that all have the right to an adequate standard of health services regardless of income, and that this right can be protected only through a programme of health services organized and administered by government. According to the Chairman of the Saskatchewan Advisory Planning Committee on Medical Care the government

cannot abdicate responsibility for an enterprise which is so large and important and which so greatly affects the national welfare and the welfare of every citizen. An enterprise which carries such great possibilities of arbitrary decisions, unequal treatment, injustice, special privileges and benefits, must be subject to the will of the electorate through the government.[2]

With the introduction of the Saskatchewan Hospital Services Plan in 1947 the economic obstacles to universal hospital care were removed.

1 / E. A. Tollefson, *Bitter Medicine*, Saskatoon: Modern Press, 1963, pp. 36–38.
2 / W. P. Thompson, *Medical Care*, Toronto: Clarke, Irwin & Co., Ltd., 1964, p. 109.

According to Roemer the inauguration of this Plan provided for a patient easy access to a doctor in a distant city,

without worry about a bigger hospital bill than would be faced in the small local hospital. In this setting it was inevitable that a prepayment plan offering free choice of doctors at any location, as well as specialist services, would provide advantages over the old municipal doctor scheme. The challenge was met by voluntary medical care insurance plans sponsored by the doctors themselves.[3]

These voluntary prepayment medical care plans sponsored by the medical profession in Saskatchewan and in other provinces may be seen, not only as an effort on the part of the profession to meet the financial hazards of sickness faced by the population, but also as an attempt by the profession to counter the rising demand by an increasingly large segment of the population for some form of government-administered universal medical care insurance. In 1948 the Swift Current Health Region, in the southwestern area of the province, was organized. This was a universal, compulsory medical care plan which provided its members with comprehensive hospital and medical services and served as a model in the subsequent development of the provincial medical care scheme.

The first of the voluntary plans in Saskatchewan, the Regina Medical Services, had been organized in 1939. As these doctor-sponsored plans developed they varied in certain respects. Medical Services Incorporated, organized in 1946, offered medical, surgical, and obstetrical benefits in the home, office, or hospital. It had three unique features:

A It pioneered the enrolment of individual persons ... B it insured the residents of whole communities under one contract; and c by arrangement with its member physicians, it ... arranged to give its beneficiaries added protection by placing controls on the extent to which its specialist member-physicians may charge the patient for specialist services, over and above the charges covered by the contract.[4]

Group Medical Services was organized in 1949, with the amalgamation of Regina Medical Services and the Group Health Association, a co-operative plan. It restricted its enrolment to groups, rather than individuals, and offered benefits similar to those of Medical Services Incorporated.

Besides these voluntary medical care insurance plans sponsored by physicians, a number of insurance companies sold accident and sickness insurance policies which reimbursed the policy holder for a stipulated

3 / Milton I. Roemer, "Prepaid Medical Care and Changing Needs in Saskatchewan," *Medical Care in Transition*, vol. I, Washington: 1964, pp. 344–50.
4 / Government of Saskatchewan, *Report of the Advisory Planning Committee on Medical Care*, Regina: Queen's Printer, 1962, pp. 17–18.

amount of the costs of physicians' and other services. In addition to these doctor-sponsored and commercial plans, a number of co-operative plans were started, but only one, the Saskatoon Mutual Medical and Hospital Benefit Association, had shown limited success in enrolling subscribers by 1960.

In that year the total number of subscribers enrolled in all these plans, plus those who were covered by other arrangements under public auspices, such as the municipal doctor plans, the Swift Current Plan, health care services for public assistance recipients, municipal aid, the armed services, and federal penitentiary inmates, equalled 67 per cent of the provincial population.[5]

These various attempts on the part of the public, the profession, the government, and the insurance industry to find some means of prepaying, in whole or in part, the costs of medical services, and sometimes a wider range of health services, were accompanied by the type of social changes noted in chapter 1: a weakening of individualist *laissez-faire* values and a strengthening of collectivist values in an increasing number of areas of human activity which affected the public's conception of the proper role of government in these matters; the urban movement of the population with the consequent difficulties in maintaining adequate levels of health facilities and personnel in rural areas; an increase in the demand for health services of the highest quality; and the rising costs of health care which were the accompaniment of technological advances in diagnosis and treatment, particularly as they affected hospital care. These changes were accompanied by others within the medical profession which have been discussed in previous chapters: the increased rate of the growth of knowledge and its technical application resulting in the proliferation of medical and paramedical specialties which affected the relationships between physicians and patients; attempts to apply new and old knowledge with a consequent pressure for a rationalization of the organization of practice, and the emergence of group practice; and attempts to maintain and possibly increase the standards of the quality of care resulting in a demand for controls of the quality of medical care.

These changes both inside and outside medicine, particularly since World War II, placed the practising physician in a difficult position. His social and professional world was changing rapidly, and many of these changes he found difficult to understand. In fact, the rate of change was so rapid that for many physicians, but particularly the non-specialists, their previous education and training in medicine appeared to offer them little support in the face of the pressures which these changes generated. There

5 / *Ibid.*, p. 26.

remained, however, certain fundamental individualist values which they had learned in medical school and which the practice of medicine appeared to support. These values were in conflict with the increasing emphasis on a collectivist ideology in many new areas of human activity, an ideology which, in Canada, had a lengthy and substantial tradition.

Conflict between the individualist and collectivist ideologies was not obvious in the early years of the CCF government, but in 1959 Premier Douglas stated that the provincial government was ready to implement a provincial programme of medical care insurance. The reaction of the profession indicated the extent of its change in attitude towards such a programme, due, in part at least, to the changes in society and in medicine noted above. At the annual meeting of the Saskatchewan College of Physicians and Surgeons in October 1959, a unanimous resolution was passed which stated, "The members of the College of Physicians and Surgeons of Saskatchewan oppose the introduction of a compulsory Government-controlled Province-wide medical care plan and declare our support of and the extension of health and sickness benefits through indemnity and services plans."[6]

In December 1959 Premier Douglas announced a plan to set up an Advisory Planning Committee on Medical Care which would report to the government on the type of medical care insurance scheme best suited to the needs of the province. This announcement was followed by lengthy negotiations between the government and the College of Physicians and Surgeons of Saskatchewan concerning membership on the committee and its terms of reference. In April 1960 the Advisory Planning Committee on Medical Care was finally set up. Later that year an election campaign was fought in the province in which one of the major issues was the type of medical care insurance the government proposed to introduce. The profession entered the electoral fray to defend its position and oppose the government proposals. According to Badgley,

"The profession had apparently studied the tactics of the American Medical Association in opposing legislative action in the United States. A tightly knit, anxious, and militant group led the profession. Doctors campaigned in all parts of the province. Copying another A.M.A. technique, a 'key man' system was set up, and each 'key man' was responsible for a small cell of doctors. Plans were passed from the profession's hierarchy to the 'key man,' then to the rank-and-file doctors. Potential medical heretics were excluded from the communications system. Public-relations experts were hired and brought in from eastern Canada."[7]

6 / Quoted in Tollefson, *Bitter Medicine*, p. 45.
7 / Robin F. Badgley and Samuel Wolfe, *Doctors' Strike*, Toronto: Macmillan Co., 1967, p. 30.

Tollefson claims that "A special voluntary levy of $100 was sought by the College of Physicians and Surgeons from each of its members to help in the campaign. Over $60,000 was collected by means of this voluntary levy. Subsequently, a gift of $35,000 was received from the Canadian Medical Association to cover any deficit."[8] Despite the campaign of the profession the CCF won the election with thirty-eight seats in the fifty-four seat provincial legislature.

In September 1961 the Advisory Planning Committee on Medical Care submitted an interim report to the government, and the final report was submitted in September 1962. The committee's major recommendations were:

1 That a medical care insurance program be established which would include the following seven basic elements:

A   Universal coverage of all residents of the province, except persons now eligible to receive direct medical (i.e. physicians') services under certain programs operated by the federal government.

B   A comprehensive range of medical service benefits, excluding services now provided under certain provincial programs.

C   Eligibility for benefits based on residence, registration and proof of payment of a medical care insurance premium.

D   A personal premium which should be at a level which can be met by all self-supporting persons, with additional financial support to be provided from the general revenues of the province.

E   Limited "utilization fees" on physicians' home and office calls, charged to insured patients at the time of service.

F   Payment for medical services to be, in general, on a fee-per-item-of-service basis, but with the provision for special methods of payment in specific situations.

G   Administration by a public commission, responsible to the government, through the Minister of Public Health.

2 That, in its financial planning, the Government take into consideration the necessity for expansion and improvement in certain other programs of health care ... These are concerned with:

A   home care,

B   rehabilitation,

C   mental health,

D   pharmaceutical services,

E   dental services,

F   continuing medical education,

G   medical research.[9]

8 / Quoted in Tollefson, *Bitter Medicine*, p. 54.

9 / Government of Saskatchewan, *Report of Advisory Planning Committee on Medical Care*, pp. 12–13.

The introduction into the legislature of the Medical Care Insurance Act, which followed closely the recommendations of the Advisory Planning Committee on Medical Care, resulted in increased criticism by physicians and their professional association. Much of this criticism was based upon the professions' interpretation of certain sections of the Act, notably section 9 and section 49 (1) particularly clauses (G) and (L). Section 9 of the Act states: "The Commission may pursuant to this Act and the regulations made by Lieutenant Governor in Council and by the commission, take such action as it considers necessary for the establishment and administration of a plan of medical care insurance for the residents of Saskatchewan and the improvement of the quality of the insured services provided under such a plan."[10]

The College interpreted the last clause in this section to mean that the Medical Care Insurance Commission was given the power to take action to raise the quality of medical care. By so doing, the Commission would be directly involved in regulating the professional behaviour of physicians. Tollefson argues that such was not the intent of this section,[11] but nevertheless the physicians of the province interpreted it as such and acted to prevent passage. Section 49 (1) and clauses (G) and (L) read as follows:

Section 49 (1) Subject to the approval of the Lieutenant Governor in Council, the commission may make regulations for the purpose of establishing and administering a plan of medical care insurance for the residents of Saskatchewan and, without restricting the generality of the foregoing may make regulations:
(G) prescribing the terms and conditions on which physicians and other persons may provide insured services to beneficiaries;
(L) respecting the maintenance and improvement of the quality of the services provided under this Act, to the end that the highest possible standards of service will be achieved.

After the Act was passed by the provincial legislature the physicians of the province reaffirmed their opposition to it. The government sought a meeting with the College of Physicians and Surgeons which the College refused for a time. In March 1962, however, both parties met, but at this and subsequent meetings the physicians maintained their objections, and were particularly unyielding in their refusal to consider the universality of the government programme, its compulsory premiums, and its administration by a government body.

On July 1, 1962, the majority of physicians in Saskatchewan withdrew

10 / The Saskatchewan Medical Care Insurance Act, 1961, Statutes of Saskatchewan, 1961 (second session), chapter 1.
11 / Tollefson, *Bitter Medicine*, p. 70.

their services after setting up an emergency service located in forty designated hospitals in the province. About seventy-five physicians continued to practise. Support for the doctors' stand was evident in the Saskatchewan press, in the provincial Liberal party, then the official opposition in the legislature, but particularly in the formation of the Keep Our Doctors committees. As the opponents of the Act became more heated in their attacks on the government, Premier Lloyd sought to avoid serious clashes between the opponents and supporters of the medical care programme by suggesting that those supporting the government's stand restrain their feelings and their public announcements.

An attempt to renew negotiations with the government was made by the College of Physicians and Surgeons on July 14, but the proposals put forward by the College were unacceptable to the government. Agreement on the points at issue in the Act was finally reached with the intervention of Lord Taylor, a British Labour peer, who had been invited to Saskatchewan by the government to act as its adviser. The physicians then accepted the universal comprehensive medical care programme proposed in the Act. The government agreed to let the existing voluntary insurance agencies collect from the government fees earned by physicians in the treatment of patients covered under the Act, and to the appointment to the Commission set up to administer the programme of three physicians, acceptable both to the profession and to the government. The dispute came to an end on July 23.

The conservative orientation of the profession affected its members' image of the government in power and their interpretation of its policies. To the average physician trained in the conservative mould of Canadian medical schools, associating with highly independent and professionally autonomous colleagues in internship, residency, and subsequent practice, and exposed to the conservative perspective of provincial and federal professional associations, the government in power in Saskatchewan was a radical party offering proposals that appeared to aim at the destruction of professional autonomy. The medical care insurance scheme of Alberta left much more discretionary power to the Minister of Public Health, but to the physicians of that province the Social Credit government was one that accorded with their own conservative values and they therefore supported its medical care legislation.

One of the reasons for the settlement of the medical care dispute in Saskatchewan was not so much a change in the attitudes of the physicians of that province towards the government in power as a clearer delineation of the government's role in the control of medical services; it was a role with which physicians did not agree but they nevertheless accepted it since sharper delineation left little room for misinterpretation. The physicians "knew where they stood" with the government, and knew the limits on the power of the Medical Care Insurance Commission. These limits were seen, in part, as a function of the increased representation of physicians on the Commission. The method of appointing physicians as members of the Commission followed an arrangement advocated by the Canadian Medical Association.[12] Regardless of the effectiveness of increased physician representation as a limitation on the power of the Commission, the fact that Saskatchewan physicians perceived this arrangement as meeting at least some of their demands created a climate in which a settlement could be reached.

In the view of the medical profession of the province the central issue in the dispute between the government and the College of Physicians and Surgeons was third-party, in this case government, control of the medical profession. Regardless of the government's claims to the contrary, once the profession had defined the situation in these terms the consequences were largely predictable. Control of the profession can be implemented through regulation of the quality, quantity, and price of medical services, and since these three variables are interdependent, regulation of one provides a degree of control over the other two.

The claims by some Saskatchewan physicians of "socialism," "statism," "dictatorship," to mention only a few, were based on traditional values of the profession which were supported by certain community-wide values, rather than on a rational evaluation of the variables involved in a degree of third-party control. The profession had, in fact, accepted a limited degree of control over price by third parties, but these were medical care prepayment plans sponsored by the profession. The proposed Saskatchewan Medical Care Insurance Act would have put these third parties out of business, and placed the responsibility for payment of medical services in the hands of the Commission which, in the final analysis, was to be responsible to the provincial legislature. Payment of physicians' fees was to become a government budgetary matter, thereby creating the possibility of government intervention in the assessment of the quality of the medical services provided by funds raised by the government.

A fundamental difficulty facing the profession and the government in Saskatchewan was to determine the mechanism which would give the latter a means of paying the physician, and at the same time guarantee the profession's control over its members and the quality of the services they provided. The importance of this issue is evident in the Memorandum of

12 / For a discussion of the manner in which the power of the Commission was curtailed see Tollefson, *Bitter Medicine*, pp. 118–32.

Agreement signed by the government and the College of Physicians and Surgeons of that province, and in the legislation amending the original Medical Care Insurance Act which settled the dispute. Tollefson shows this importance statistically:

The main body of the Saskatoon Agreement contains twenty-nine articles. Of these, a total of fourteen could be classified as being statements of belief or general policy, and nine deal with questions relating to payment for insured services. In the remaining six articles, only the matter of the Medical Care Insurance Commission receives treatment in more than one article. Similarly, more than one-half of the amending legislation is devoted to setting out the law relating to payment for insured services.[13]

The agreement between the government and the profession resulted in the maintenance of the existing physician-sponsored third-party arrangements, designated as "approved health agencies," whose sole purpose under the amended legislation is to pay physicians' bills for services rendered. Two other possible arrangements were agreed upon: direct payment to physicians for their services to insured patients by the Medical Care Insurance Commission and payment to the patient by the Commission of an amount equal to an agreed proportion of the profession's schedule of fees. If a physician wishes to practise outside these arrangements he is free to do so. The administrative expenses of the approved health agencies are raised through a premium on their members. Services other than those offered under the Saskatchewan Medical Care Insurance Act may be offered by these approved agencies for an additional premium cost. In effect these bodies have become collection agencies and provide no protection to physicians using their services from government control and regulation. The control of standards of medical care still legally rests with the College of Physicians and Surgeons, a right delegated by statute by the legislature, but it is a legislature now with a concern for the costs of medical care which can result in a concern with quality.

The Saskatchewan Medical Care Insurance Plan has been in operation for five years. In that time the Liberal party has come to power in the province, a party which supported the physicians during their dispute with the former CCF government. This change in government may be associated with some change in the attitudes of physicians in the province towards the Plan, but if such a change in attitudes of individual physicians has occurred it may not be shared by functionaries of the College of Physicians and Surgeons of that province. This is evident in the attempt by W. P. Thompson, a former Professor of Genetics, President Emeritus of the University

13 / *Ibid.*, p. 123.

of Saskatchewan, and Chairman of the Advisory Planning Committee on Medical Care which laid the ground work for the original Medical Care Insurance legislation, to undertake a survey of the opinions of Saskatchewan physicians regarding the effects of the medical care legislation after it had been in force for three years. While the survey was underway the Council of the College of Physicians and Surgeons sent a letter to physicians in the province claiming that the questionnaire used in the survey was open to serious criticism.[14] This action on the part of the College makes impossible the task of determining the extent of changes in physicians' attitudes toward the Saskatchewan Medical Care Insurance Plan since its inception from the data derived from this survey. Furthermore there is no reliable measure of this attitude prior to the introduction of the Saskatchewan Plan.

One can assume that if conditions had remained the same in Saskatchewan, that is, if the provision of medical care insurance by third parties had not been taken over by government as its responsibility, physicians' attitudes towards government-administered medical care insurance would have changed slowly, if at all, in a more favourable direction. But conditions of practice in Saskatchewan changed in spite of the College's attempts to prevent them, and physicians found themselves practising under conditions they had claimed would be against their interests and those of their patients.

Did this situation create more favourable attitudes towards the Saskatchewan Plan on the part of physicians practising in that province? A conclusive answer to this question is not possible with available data, but recent material published by the Saskatchewan Medical Care Insurance Commission suggests that such a change may be occurring gradually. As indicated earlier, the agreement of July 1962 which settled the dispute between the College of Physicians and Surgeons and the Government contained three methods of fee-for-service payment for insured services: a direct payment by the Commission to the physician on submission of a bill for services rendered; payment through an approved health agency, the physician submitting his bill to the agency which, in turn, submits it to the Commission and receives payment from the Commission, and then forwards payment to the physician; and payment by the Commission to the patient for insured services. The direct payment was the method to which the profession took strong objections since it involved a direct financial relationship between physician and government which the profession believed could lead to interference and control of the former by the latter.

14 / W. P. Thompson, "Saskatchewan Doctors' Opinions of 'Medicare,' " *Canadian Medical Association Journal*, vol. 93, October 30, 1965, pp. 971–76.

Despite the profession's initial negative attitude towards this method of payment a gradually increasing proportion of Saskatchewan physicians has used the direct payment method. In 1963, the year following the introduction of the Plan, 21.1 per cent of all claims received by the Commission were forwarded directly by the physicians; by 1967 this figure reached 36.4 per cent. Claims received by the Commission from health agencies, although increasing in number, decreased in percentage terms from 68.1 to 59.4, and claims received from patients decreased from 10.8 per cent to 4.2 per cent.[15] These data may reflect a more favourable attitude towards the Saskatchewan Plan by an increasing percentage of physicians in that province. This change may have developed as the inconsistency between the fears on which their negative attitude was based and the realities of practice under the Plan became obvious with the passage of time.

As noted earlier the quality, quantity, and costs of medical care are interrelated. Today, provincial and federal governments are assuming increasing responsibility for the costs of medical care through government sponsored or administered medical care insurance, and for the amount of medical care through the provision of medical education facilities and the supply of physicians. These developments place the medical profession in a relationship with government closer than it has experienced in the past, and one which may create concern by government with the quality of medical care. Unless the legislature is satisfied that the existing professional control mechanisms are effective in maintaining quality, it will create some other means. This emerging situation places the medical profession under severe pressure to create a control structure which can maintain high standards of medical care. Despite their claims of antipathy towards government intereference and control in professional matters, the changes in certain conditions of practice, which are now evident in Saskatchewan and which will emerge with the introduction of government-sponsored medical care insurance in other provinces, could bring about a profound change in attitudes towards quality control.

THE ROYAL COMMISSION ON HEALTH SERVICES

The seven members of the Commission were appointed by the Progressive Conservative government in 1961 to study and report upon the whole range of health services in Canada, to determine future needs, and the resources required to meet them. The Commission was also charged "to recommend such measures consistent with the constitutional division of

15 / Saskatchewan, Medical Care Insurance Commission, *Annual Report*, 1964, 1967.

legislative powers in Canada, as the Commissioners believe will ensure that *the best possible health care is available to all Canadians.*"[16] In February 1964 the Commission, minus one of its members who had been appointed to the Senate of Canada, submitted volume I of its Final Report to the Liberal government of the day. In December 1964, volume II of the Final Report was submitted. The most significant recommendation of the Commission was the development of a comprehensive health services programme universally available to all Canadians regardless of age, condition, place of residence, or ability to pay for services. The programme was to cover not only medical care services, but the whole range of personal health services including prescribed drugs, dental and optical services for children and public assistance recipients, organized care for crippled and mentally retarded children, prosthetic services, home care services, the reorganization of the mental health services of the nation, and important changes in the existing hospital insurance programme. The underlying concern of the Commission was the gap which existed between scientific knowledge and skills in the field of health and the ability of the society to apply them to all who need them. In the words of the Commission: *"What the Commission recommends is that in Canada this gap be closed. That as a nation we now take the necessary legislative, organizational and financial decisions to make all the fruits of the health sciences available to all our residents without hindrance of any kind. All our recommendations are directed towards this objective."*[17]

The Commissioners recognized that many Canadians had availed themselves of the benefits of health prepayment plans, but these were principally those who could afford protection or were employed where health insurance was provided or subsidized as a part of working conditions. They concluded that coverage of all, or virtually all, Canadians could not be achieved through the voluntary system and that only a universal programme could achieve maximum coverage. In order to spread the risks over the whole population rather than only those who chose to insure voluntarily, all Canadians should be covered by health insurance. The Commissioners rejected all methods of subsidizing individuals that involve means testing on the grounds that the proportion of the population to be means tested would be too large and the administrative costs too high. In addition they were of the view that such testing is not in accord with human dignity. Instead they recommended that a health insurance fund be established in each province, contributed to by the federal govern-

16 / Royal Commission on Health Services, *Final Report*, vol. I, p. x (italics in original).
17 / *Ibid.*, p. 10 (italics in original).

ment from general revenue and by the provincial government from premiums, sales, or other taxes or general revenues. It was the belief of the Commissioners that such a fund, when established by democratically elected legislatures, with outlays limited to the essentials of health care, with citizens having free choice of physicians, and able to insure additional items of health services through private organizations, could not be said to be compulsory in any democratic sense of the term. Rather, according to the Commission, democratic ideals would be more fully realized.

The Commission was confident that the medical needs of all Canadians could be met through the prepayment system it proposed. Its confidence was based on the fact that the proposals of the Canadian Medical Association and the Canadian Health Insurance Association, contained in their respective briefs to the Commission, indicated that the medical profession was capable of meeting the medical needs of all Canadians on a prepayment basis. The Commission therefore assumed that if spokesmen for the medical profession were confident that it could meet all the needs of Canadians when they were insured through profession-sponsored prepayment plans and the insurance industry, then there should be no less confidence in the ability of the profession to meet these needs under the programme recommended by the Commission where the only difference was how the programme was to be financed and services paid for.

The Commission maintained that under its recommended programme the freedom of the physician and the patient would be protected. In the Commission's words:

The most fundamental feature of the programmes recommended is that they are based on free, independent, self-governing professions. The provision of and payment for services is to be the result of a negotiated contractual relationship based principally on the fee-for-service concept. The physician continues in private practice. He renders the service which, in his judgment, his diagnosis indicates. The state does not interfere in any way with his professional management of the patient's condition, nor with the confidential nature of the physician-patient relationship.[18]

In answer to those physicians, and their representatives and others, who claimed that the introduction of a universal, comprehensive prepaid health services programme would result in a deterioration in the quality of medical care, the Commission pointed out that since there appeared to be no such claim providing individuals were universally insured under a physician-sponsored medical care prepayment plan there was no necessary reason why such a claim should be valid if the programme was sponsored by government. Furthermore, the Commission pointed out that it had

18 / *Ibid.*, vol. II, p. 10.

recommended substantial assistance for medical students and graduates plus programmes for the building of new medical schools and the expansion of existing ones in order to increase the number of physicians. The Commission also suggested that the introduction of universal medical care would attract more physicians and educate the public to the importance of early preventive treatment and that both these developments would improve the quality of medical care.

As for the costs of its recommended programme the Commission contended that Canada could afford the required financial outlays. Studies prepared for the Commission showed that Canada's economic growth would be sufficient to provide the funds required, and that these funds would fulfil the function of investment as well as of consumption. Despite the large and growing expenditures on health care they had not been out of line with the growth of Canadian income. Much of the postwar increase in spending on health care was due to the re-establishment of a pattern of spending that had been seriously disrupted by the depression of the 1930s and World War II. The rate of spending on health care in recent years had thus reflected a "catching up" process in this area. In this period health expenditures had continued to grow more rapidly than either income or consumer spending beause of the changes occurring in the manner of financing health care such as the growth of prepaid medical care programmes and the hospital insurance programme. The Commission pointed out, however, that despite the increase in public spending for health care, the construction of health facilities, health research, and the education of health personnel, expenditures on health care amounted to only 5.4 per cent of Gross National Expenditure in 1961. This could be compared with 4.5 per cent to 5.5 per cent of Gross National Expenditure then being spent for this purpose by most western nations.

The Commission estimated that a continuation of the present system of health services, with its limitations and inadequacies, would cost $4,015 million annually or $178 per person, but for an additional $466 million or $20 per person Canada could have the universal, comprehensive programme recommended by the Commission.

RECENT DEVELOPMENTS

The introduction and evidently successful operation of medical care insurance in Saskatchewan and the far-reaching recommendations of the Royal Commission on Health Services were two developments which strengthened the collectivist ideology of medical care. In the House of Commons all parties hailed the Commission's Report as an important social document. Some form of government universal comprehensive medical care insurance in all provinces seemed inevitable.

In 1965 following the Report of the Royal Commission on Health Services, the federal government laid down four criteria which provincial medical care plans had to meet if they were to receive federal financial assistance. These criteria were: (1) coverage and benefits under the provincial plans should be portable from province to province, (2) the plan should be publicly administered and accountable, (3) all services rendered by physicians should be covered, and (4) the plans should cover all eligible population.

These were incorporated into the 1966 Medical Care Act in the following terms:

4 1 A medical care insurance plan of a province in respect of which a contribution is payable by Canada to the province for a year pursuant to section 3 is a plan, established pursuant to an Act of the legislature of the province (hereinafter referred to as the "provincial law"), that throughout the year satisfies the following criteria:

A the plan is administered and operated on a non-profit basis by a public authority appointed or designated by the government of the province (hereinafter referred to as the "provincial authority"), that is responsible in respect of the administration and operation of the plan to the government of the province or to a provincial minister designated by the government of the province for such purpose, and that is subject in respect of its accounts and financial transactions to audit by such person as is charged by law with the audit of the accounts of the province;

B the plan provides for and is administered and operated so as to provide for the furnishing of insured services upon uniform terms and conditions to all insurable residents of the province, by the payment of amounts in respect of the cost of insured services in accordance with a tariff of authorized payments established pursuant to the provincial law or in accordance with any other system of payment authorized by the provincial law, on a basis that provides for reasonable compensation for insured services rendered by medical practitioners and that does not impede or preclude, either directly or indirectly whether by charges made to insured persons or otherwise, reasonable access to insured services by insured persons;

C the number of insurable residents of the province who are entitled under the plan to insured services is not less than 90% of the total number of insurable residents of the province, except that in applying this paragraph for the purpose of determining whether the plan satisfies the criteria set forth in this subsection throughout the third and each subsequent year after the year commencing on the contribution commencement day, there shall be substituted for the expression "90%" in this paragraph the expression "95%"; and

D the plan does not impose any minimum period of residence in the province or any waiting period in excess of three months before persons who are or become residents of the province are eligible for or entitled to insured services, and the plan provides for and is administered and operated so as to provide for the payment of amounts in respect of the cost of insured services furnished to insured persons while temporarily absent from the province, and in the case of persons who have ceased to be insured persons by reason of having become residents of another participating province, of the cost of insured services furnished to such persons during any minimum period of residence or waiting period imposed by the medical care insurance plan of that other province, on the same basis as though such persons had not been absent from the province or had not ceased to be residents of the province, as the case may be.[19]

The introduction of government universal medical care insurance in Saskatchewan in 1962, the Report of the Royal Commission on Health Services in 1964, and the resulting federal Medical Care Act of 1966 were accompanied by the development of a pattern of medical care insurance in a number of other provinces. One province, Alberta, had already indicated prior to the publication of the Report of the Royal Commission that although publicly operated medical care programmes might be unavoidable the extent to which the provincial government became involved could be limited.

The Social Credit party of Alberta had emerged as the government of that province in a period of drought and depression. Its success at the polls was due to the protest of low income groups against their economically depressed status. The coalition of fundamentalist religion and the Social Credit party, personified in Premier Aberhart, was

a reaction against the forces of urbanism, cultural maturity, and centralization both economic and religious, and a defence of past traditions and mores: of the rural against the urban, and of the cultural independence of immigrant ethnic groups ... the very vigour and scope of its protest acted as a corrective to insistent economic forces of urbanization, centralization, and uniformity that tended to twist and uproot deep-lying traditions and symbolic systems.[20]

This anti-centralist and anti-collectivist tradition is carried on today, in a somewhat modified form, by the present Social Credit government of the province whose leader until the end of 1968, Premier Manning, used

19 / Statutes of Canada, 14–15 Elizabeth II, chapter 64, Medical Care Act, section 4.
20 / W. E. Mann, "Sect and Cult in Western Canada," in B. R. Blishen *et al.* (eds.), *Canadian Society*, 2nd ed., Toronto: Macmillan Co., 1964, pp. 365–66.

both his clerical and his political roles to condemn the collectivist trend and promote the free enterprise ideology of medical care. A government with these views could not be expected to agree to a universal medical care plan under which everybody was covered for the payment of physicians' fees regardless of income. Therefore, the government of Alberta introduced its own Medical Plan in 1963, which authorized it to subsidize those individuals wishing to be covered under the Plan but whose incomes were too low to permit them to pay the premiums of the physician-sponsored and commercial insurance companies. The Alberta Medical Plan thus authorized the Minister of Health of the Province to:

A ... enter into agreements with Medical Services (Alberta) Incorporated or any insurance corporation whose basic programme of prepaid medical services or medical services insurance has been approved by the Government and the College of Physicians and Surgeons of the Province of Alberta to make available prepaid medical services or medical services insurance with comprehensive benefits to those eligible residents who desire it and need assistance to purchase the contracts provided by that corporation and to provide a specified dollar subsidy in respect of those residents who need assistance on the condition that the cost of the prepayment premium or insurance to those residents is reduced by the amount of the subsidy.[21]

The intent of the Plan was to attain universal coverage of the population of the province without compulsion through the payment of premiums, subsidized from public funds, to approved private insurance carriers offering comprehensive physicians' services in home, office, and hospital. The individual was free to buy medical care insurance if he wanted to and could afford it, or to apply for government subsidy if he could not pay the insurance premiums. In this manner the myth of "free enterprise" medical care was maintained. In 1966 the Plan was supplemented with the inclusion, for an additional premium, of health benefits other than physicians' services, but it also included provision for a deductible amount, or co-insurance which requires the insured to pay a specified proportion of the cost of the services received, plus limited financial liability of the insurer on certain services. The government agreed to pay 80 per cent of the cost of the premiums for subscribers who reported no taxable income for the previous year, 50 per cent of the cost of the premiums for those whose taxable income was from $1 to $499, and 25 per cent of the cost of the premiums for those whose taxable income was from $500 to $1000. In 1967 this Plan was superseded by one in which a government agency, rather than physician-sponsored or commercial medical care insurance

21 / Amendment to the Treatment Services Act, Revised Statutes of Alberta, 1963, 14th Legislature, 5th session.

plans, was responsible for voluntary enrolment and for the payment of physicians' fees for services rendered under the new scheme. The premiums under this Plan are $60 a year for single persons, $120 a year for two-person families, and $160 a year for families of three persons or more. For families with less than $1000 taxable income, and for single persons with less than $500 taxable income in the previous year premium reductions range from 90 per cent to 66 per cent.[22]

Plans similar to that in Alberta in 1967 have been set up in British Columbia and Ontario. In both provinces the governments, the physicians, and the insurance companies have claimed that this method of providing medical care maintains the traditions of free enterprise since other voluntary enrolment medical care insurance plans sponsored by provincial physicians' associations, commercial insurance companies, or independent groups continue to exist alongside the government plans. The British Columbia Medical Plan went into operation in 1965 and is administered by a government agency whose direction is controlled by representatives of both the government and the medical profession and is responsible for enrolment, collection of premiums, and the payment of physicians' claims. Premiums under the Plan are $60 annually for single persons, $120 for a two-person family, and $150 for a family of three or more. For persons with no taxable income and for persons with a taxable income of $1 to $1000 the Plan offers premium reductions ranging from 90 per cent to 50 per cent.[23]

The Ontario Medical Services Insurance Plan which began operation in 1966 is administered by a government agency with the responsibility for enrolment, collection of premiums, and the payment of physicians' claims. Annual premiums are the same as those of the British Columbia Medical Plan. For those unable to pay the cost of the premium the Plan pays 50 per cent of the premium for single applicants who have taxable incomes of $500 or less; 50 per cent for families of two persons with a taxable income of $1000 or less; and 60 per cent of the premium for families of three or more persons with a taxable income of $1300 or less.[24]

After the introduction of the federal Medical Care Act in 1966 the provincial governments of Alberta, British Columbia, and Ontario sought to meet the criteria specified in the Act in the organization of their respective medical care insurance plans while maintaining voluntary participation as a basic feature in order to meet the opposition of the spokesmen

22 / Canada, Department of National Health and Welfare, *Provincial Health Services by Program*, Ottawa: 1968, p. 172.
23 / *Ibid.*, p. 175.
24 / *Ibid.*, p. 174.

for the medical profession who claim that government-administered, universal, medical care plans would create an increased demand for physicians' services which could not be met without a greatly increased supply of physicians. As noted previously, the Royal Commission on Health Services questioned the validity of this claim by pointing out that the medical profession made no such claim providing a universal plan was based on voluntary participation without government administration.

The introduction of universal medical care insurance which is administered and controlled by government or sponsored by physicians or commercial firms and which is not accompanied by an increase in the supply of physicians, and possibly some reorganization of the manner in which their services are delivered, results in role strains for physicians due to the increased utilization of their services. The physician may reap substantial financial benefits from such a situation as Berry points out. He estimates the average payments to individual physicians under a universal medical care scheme and compares them with the average gross income of physicians in private practice in 1961. The results for some provinces are startling. In Newfoundland the payments under universal medical care are $52,911 compared with an average gross income in 1961 of $22,412; in Prince Edward Island the comparison is between $32,503 and $20,229; in Nova Scotia between $31,369 and $23,123 and New Brunswick between $37,032 and $23,991. In other provinces the differences were not as great.[25] Regardless of the type of plan, government or voluntary, there can be little doubt that in this situation of increased demand for physicians' services plus the economic incentives for the physicians to attempt to meet it, the pressure to lower standards of medical care would be difficult for the individual physician to avoid, but under a government plan the relaxation of quality would bring into operation the control procedures of the government administrative agency. Such procedures could be more restrictive of professional autonomy than those applied by the voluntary physician-sponsored plans which the physician now accepts. The issue of control is crucial for the professional independence and status of organized medicine, an issue that was an important consideration in the recommendations of the Royal Commission on Health Services regarding the organization of medical services.[26]

The Commission suggested that each province agreeing to a universal health services programme should set up a provincial health services commission in which the public, the health professions, and the government

25 / C. H. Berry, *Voluntary Medical Insurance and Prepayment*, Royal Commission on Health Services, Ottawa: Queen's Printer, 1964, p. 167.
26 / Royal Commission on Health Services, *Final Report*, vol. II, pp. 199–200.

are represented and which should be responsible for the planning, evaluation, and administration of health services in the province. The Commission should report to the legislature through the Minister of Health.[27] Physicians, and other health services personnel, would retain their respective responsibilities for providing professional services, but payment for their services would come from the provincial Commission. This Commission, however, would be responsible to the provincial legislature to which it would report its activities annually.[28]

It is this legislative control through a provincial commission with which the medical profession disagrees for it fears that control of the payment mechanism might be used to impose conditions of practice which would restrict professional autonomy by possibly setting up a review of the manner in which services are provided and by questioning the quality of care and its cost. Final budgetary control would lie with the legislature, and such control might be used to question the behaviour of physicians. This possibility was not overlooked by the Royal Commission on Health Services which attempted to provide safeguards for the professional autonomy of the physicians participating in its recommended universal medical care insurance scheme. Nevertheless, it recognized the ultimate power of the democratically elected legislature: "Organized medicine is a statutory creation of legislatures and of parliament. When the state grants a monopoly to an exclusive group to render an indispensable service it automatically becomes involved in whether those services are available and on what terms and conditions."[29]

Despite the continuing fears of the medical profession of government intervention in professional matters, two provinces, British Columbia and Saskatchewan, signed an agreement in 1968 with the federal government under the Medical Care Act. In the same year Manitoba, Nova Scotia, and Newfoundland expressed their intention of coming into the federal plan, and New Brunswick discussed with the federal government the financial implications of implementing the federal plan in that province.

As provinces move to develop medical care insurance plans which meet the conditions laid down in the Medical Care Act the costs of medical care continue to rise sharply. Two of the major factors affecting the cost of medical care, physicians' fees and the volume of care provided, have risen substantially in all provinces in the past few years. Between 1965 and 1967 the appropriate professional body in every province up-dated the physicians' fee schedule resulting in a significant rise in this element

27 / *Ibid.*, p. 215.
28 / *Ibid.*
29 / *Ibid.*, p. 11.

in the price of medical care. A provincial government medical care insurance plan could introduce controls to reduce the rate of increase in physicians' fees. The volume of care provided by physicians has increased by about 4.4 per cent per year in the period 1966 to 1968, and the possibility exists that this rate of increase will continue at least for the short run, with the introduction of government medical care insurance plans in every province. But some part of this increase may be due to the provision of unnecessary medical services because the provincial plan will be paying the physicians' fees. With rising fees and volume of care the possibility of some form of cost control at the provincial level, with its resulting controls for both the manner in which medical services are delivered, and the quality of these services, seems inevitable. Thus the fears of the medical profession of government control over some essential elements of present-day medical practice may be realized.

9

THE FOUNDATIONS OF
IDEOLOGY

THE IDEOLOGY of a profession can be derived from official statements by the organization representing the profession concerning issues which affect the professional status of its members. As noted in chapter 2 the ideology will contain ideas, values, and beliefs concerning the nature of the professional role, its relationship to other social roles, and to the society. When the profession faces change, or when its members are under attack, it will emphasize these ideas, values, and beliefs in its official statements. These elements in its ideology are evident in the statements of the Canadian Medical Association as it sought to protect the interests of its members facing the possible introduction of government-sponsored health and medical care insurance during the past twenty-five years. This is not to say that particular statements which are part of the content of the ideology are true or false. Some of these statements are judgments based on value premises which physicians share with other members of Canadian society, but certain segments of the ideology containing these values are apparently inconsistent or in conflict. In other words, the medical ideology, like other ideologies, is not a neatly articulated web of mutually compatible statements. Some inconsistent strands do exist, and may make the observer wonder how the medical profession and the individual physician can hold such incompatible, and sometimes opposing premises. Sociologists have shown that some social roles are supported by beliefs that are incompatible or in conflict with the beliefs which support other roles, but this does not necessarily lead to anxiety and strain within the individual. For example, a person's social roles, including his occupational and professional roles, are performed in a sequence; they are separated by time as well as by place. In these instances, then, the incompatibilities are insulated from each other.[1]

1 / For a discussion of these factors see especially Robert K. Merton, *Social Theory and Social Structure*, rev. and enlarged ed., Glencoe, Ill.: The Free Press, 1957, pp. 371–79.

THE GENESIS OF IDEOLOGY

The ideological beliefs of the medical profession have emerged out of the common Canadian cultural heritage. This heritage embraces mutually compatible ideological elements whose genesis can be observed in the historical development of Canadian society.

One of the most important features of Canadian social development was the rejection of the idea of revolution, specifically the American Revolution. By 1774, the northern colonies seemed bound to be embroiled in the coming revolution, if not on one side, then on the other. But though they had their political grievances like those of the Thirteen Colonies, the lack of communal feeling among people separated by geography, ethnic affiliation, and class proved insurmountable barriers to the revolutionary impetus.

The rejection by the northern colonies of revolution as an answer to national problems was strengthened by the suppression of the revolutionary idea in Upper and Lower Canada in 1837. Henceforth, political policy was aimed at building a unified economy. The problems involved in pursuing this goal, combined with the fear of United States expansion and encroachments, led to Confederation in 1867. Canadians now had the authority and resources necessary to attempt a transcontinental dominion. Self-government had come to Canada as the culmination of an evolutionary process of administrative changes instituted by colonial officials in the face of the constant threat from its southern neighbour.

The rejection of the American experiment left Canadians with no alternative but to support existing social institutions, with their built-in historical biases, including a belief in gradualism, in evolution rather than revolution; in a monarchical tradition embodied in Parliament; in peace, order, and good government; in convention and tradition; and in diversity.

The conservative tone of traditional Canadian institutions was strengthened during the development of the frontier. Canada could not leave its frontier communities exposed and unprotected against the expansionist tendencies of its southern neighbour. The North West Mounted Police, by maintaining law and order in new communities, reinforced the respect for these institutions to the extent that the population was not under pressure to take the law into its own hands through mob action.

A significant feature of Canada's cultural heritage is her dependency status. For example, Canadian economic development from its earlier beginnings has manifested a dependence on external support. Canada's economy after 1867 was based on natural resources and geographic environment. These resources were rich but the country was one of vast distances, forbidding climate, and sparse population. Development was dependent on large-scale investment from abroad. Canada retained economic as well as political ties with Britain, and, most significant for its future economic independence, it was faced with the tremendous competitive power of the United States. The dependent nature of the economy and problems posed by geographic environment required collective action if economic development was to be sustained. Such an approach to national problems was evident in the development of the Canadian Pacific Railway. The generous government financial assistance given to this venture was repeated in a later era during the building of the Canadian Northern and Grand Trunk railways. When these two enterprises seemed about to collapse for lack of financial resources, the government took them over to form the basis of a state-owned transportation system. These factors not only created support for a belief in collective action under certain circumstances, a belief that still prevails, but they also brought home to Canadians the fact that they could not obtain the heights of individual economic achievement which were evident in the United States. Individual achievement there was, of course, but its scope was much restricted compared with that to the south, and those who were fortunate enough to amass great riches generally required the overt and sometimes covert support of government to gain their ends.

From this Canadian cultural heritage, stamped in the mould of historical experience, have emerged certain beliefs and values, some of which have been noted above. When one seeks to describe them one finds that they seem to be between those of the United States and those of Britain. In a sense, both these countries serve English Canadians as examples of what they are, or what they would like to be, and what they are not. At times both these models are used in a positive manner and in other situations in a negative fashion. More specifically, the United States is preferred as an example of the opportunities and openness of society, of the extent to which equalitarian values can permeate human relationships. But this model is constrained by that of Britain with its greater emphasis on elitism. In comparison with the United States, therefore, the expression of equalitarianism is more muted in Canada.

The United States serves as the model for the amenities of daily living and for a standard of success based upon a drive to excel in a competitive but equal struggle with one's fellows. The emphasis on achievement exemplified in this model is constrained by the more elitist characteristics of that of Britain. As Lipset points out, Canada lies between these two countries in the emphasis on achievement. For evidence he provides data on the differences between the three countries in the opportunities for advancement through higher education. He shows that for the age cohort twenty to twenty-four, the United States has almost seven times the proportion enrolled in institutions of higher learning than has England and Wales. In Canada, the proportion is more than double that of England and Wales but less than a third of that of the United States. He also shows that these differences "reflect variation in values, and not simply differences in wealth and occupational structures."[2]

In the United States there is a cultivation of openness and change, and a dislike of order, a consequence of the emphasis on equality and achievement. "Hope lies in the future. Much of life becomes a preparation for some next stage where one is more competent, wealthier, freer, more secure, or more powerful."[3] In Canada there is less commitment to change, and a greater respect for order. "There seems to be less optimism, less faith in the future, less willingness to risk capital or reputation. Compared to the United States, Canada is a country of greater caution, reserve, and restraint."[4] It is similar to the English model which stands for stability, public dignity, and order.

In Canada this hesitancy in the face of change is related to the practice of "brokerage politics," in which political parties seek to balance the gains and losses in power inherent in the compromises required by conflicting interests. Canada is a pluralist society in which a large number of stable and independent groups represent many different, and sometimes conflicting, interests. This society functions as a system of checks and balances in which the opposing groups operate as countervailing forces restraining each others' powers. These groups represent economic, political, religious, ethnic, scientific, professional, and other interests. Canadian political parties have sought to create a national consensus among these competing interest groups by giving to each some part of its demands so that its members will be disposed to reward the party for its largesse. In this system of "brokerage politics" the medical profession has played its part with its claims for the protection of what it conceives to be the legitimate interests of its members.

Canadians like to think that they believe in progress, but they are not addicted to change for its own sake especially when this means that hard-won compromises may be threatened. On the other hand, despite the respect for order, caution, and restraint, there is a belief in diversity, in a cultural mosaic, although this is restrained by a basic dichotomy between

2 / S. M. Lipset, *The First New Nation*, New York: Basic Books, Inc., 1963, pp. 259–61.

3 / Kaspar D. Naegele, "Canadian Society: Further Reflections," in B. R. Blishen *et al.* (eds.), *Canadian Society*, 2nd ed., Toronto: Macmillan Co., 1964, p. 498.

4 / *Ibid.*, p. 501.

the English and French cultures. Furthermore, the relative lack of optimism and faith in the future when compared with the United States is offset to some extent by the belief that the future is full of promises of greater wealth and a larger population; yet this belief fails to generate excitement. This lack of excitement – the inability of the majority to become vitally involved in national issues – is due to the pluralist character of Canadian society with its provincial, regional, cultural, economic, parochial, sectarian, and other interests which seem to bite more deeply.

These few examples of Canadian values provide some indication of their muted character, and of their indistinctiveness. The values are there but they are so muted or blurred that public policies must be essentially pragmatic, attempting to balance a variety of competing interests, and maintaining the diversity of ethnic and regional cultures. Nevertheless, as the Canadian cultural heritage has developed, certain values, however indistinct, have emerged which provide the basic value framework within which legitimate existing ideologies must be contained. These values are not uniquely Canadian; they are shared with western democratic nations, but particularly with Britain and the United States. Canada's former economic, military, and political dependence on Britain created a value climate in which people were committed "to pursue and support certain *directions* or types of action for the collectivity as a system and hence derivatively for their own roles in the collectivity."[5] Some of the predominantly British values – which is not to say they are not also evident in the United States – are "justice," "freedom," "order," "security," "individual responsibility," and "public responsibility." Similarly, because of the high degree of Canada's economic dependence on the United States, their close geographical proximity with its consequence for easy and intensive communication, certain predominantly American values, "equality," "opportunity," "achievement," "success," and "progress," values which are, of course, also evident in Britain, have become part of Canadian culture.

The ideologies of professional or interest groups, including medicine, must be contained within this basic value framework. Sharp differences in value emphasis between ideologies are, however, sometimes evident. Sutton, for instance, contrasts the American business ideology with that of labour:

The symbols of democracy – political and religious freedom, equality of opportunity, and progress – have been accepted by all the major American ideologies. It is rather in the matter of emphasis that ideologies differ, and here these differences are great and conspicuous. The contrasts between the business

5 / Talcott Parsons, *Structure and Process in Modern Societies*, Glencoe, Ill.: The Free Press, 1960, p. 172.

ideology and the ideology of labour unions on such symbols as security, adventure, self-reliance, and productivity provide an obvious example. The business creed certainly does not assert that security is a bad thing, any more than labour unions deny the virtues of self-reliance.[6]

Since Canada, like other highly industrialized societies, is characterized by a proliferation of occupations and professions which create a socially heterogeneous environment, the ideological beliefs of one profession or social group will tend to be different in certain respects when compared with those of another. Social heterogeneity creates a difference in ideological beliefs which is a basis of controversy. Besides the social difference generated by a pattern of industrialization which it shares with a number of other nations, Canada has its tradition of social and cultural differentiation based on ethnic, religious, regional, and other interests referred to earlier. These social differences make ideological consensus difficult.

Social homogeneity within any one group is reflected in the similarity of group beliefs. As indicated previously,[7] among physicians there is a high degree of similarity of class background with the highest proportion coming from families in the upper socio-economic classes. Since beliefs to some extent are inherited from one's family, this similarity in class background will create conditions for a similarity of beliefs. This possibility will increase as class and other characteristics of social background become more homogeneous. The high degree of occupational inheritance in medicine means that a significant proportion of physicians will learn the appropriate medical ideology in the home even before entering the profession. This early indoctrination will make for stability of beliefs in later life.[8] Furthermore, a high degree of social homogeneity, as in the medical profession, also means that beliefs will be held with high intensity. This probability is evident in the medical profession's reaction to what it sees as a threat to its belief in professional freedom and autonomy. The uniformity in the claims of physicians concerning the necessity for such freedom and autonomy and the intensity with which this belief is proclaimed are related to the degree of social homogeneity in the profession as well as to the profession's conception of the importance of the issue to its survival.

The ideology of organized medicine in Canada is generally linked with basic Canadian values, but in some instances the values upon which its official policy appears to be based seem to diverge sharply from the

6 / Francis X. Sutton *et al.*, *The American Business Creed*, Cambridge, Mass.: Harvard University Press, 1956, p. 285.

7 / See Tables 2 and 3.

8 / Bernard Berelson and Gary A. Steiner, *Human Behaviour: An Inventory of Scientific Findings*, New York: Harcourt, Brace and World, Inc., 1964, p. 564.

prevailing Canadian social ideology. This divergence, however, may be more apparent than real for, as noted above, typically Canadian values are indistinct and blurred, thus making comparison of them with professional or other ideologies a difficult, if not impossible, task in some instances. The indistinctness also provides the conditions for conflict between endemic social ideologies. In other words, when beliefs and values to which differing ideologies can be allied are not clearly defined, the differences between professional and other ideologies and the central value framework of the society will tend to grow and make a dialogue between them difficult.

THE DEVELOPMENT OF
THE IDEOLOGY OF MEDICAL CARE

The nature and development of a particular professional ideology can be studied by analysing that profession's reactions to the changing conditions of work. The themes, propositions, and professional values which are embedded in the medical ideology can thus, on the one hand, be related to the role strains with which the physician must come to terms, and on the other to the heritage of values already described. The physician reacts to the strains of his role by compulsively and vigorously asserting the basic themes and professional values of the medical ideology in terms which indicate that he defines his activities as morally acceptable according to societal values.

The ideological beliefs, themes, and values to be discussed on the following pages will be analyzed as the reactions of physicians to the strains they face in the performance of their professional role. This is not to suggest that all physicians will react in the same way; some will react to role strains with a set of ideological beliefs which will not agree in some respects with those held by others, but it is a major theoretical assumption of this analysis that the strains facing the physicians today are common to most of them, and that, apart from individual idiosyncracies in reaction to strain, their reactions will be similar.

The connection between the medical profession's reaction to the strains in the roles of its members and its ideology is most obvious in its stand on health insurance in general and medical care insurance in particular. That ideology is particularly evident in the official statements of principles governing the profession's stand on this matter by the Canadian Medical Association and its provincial branches. The analysis which follows will be limited to the official statements of the national association.[9] But before

9 / The periodic statements of the Canadian Medical Association on health and medical care insurance were obtained from the Association, and are contained in appendices I to VI.

analysing the content of this ideology in terms of these strains a brief chronological review of the development of the ideology is in order.

The Canadian Medical Association has consistently maintained the view that it should not recommend a national health insurane plan, but that it should state principles upon which any such plan should be based. The first such statement of principles by the Association was released in 1934. These were periodically re-examined, and in 1943 at a special meeting the General Council of the Canadian Medical Association approved "the adoption of the principle of health insurance."[10] Its resolution, although clearly stating the Association's general approval of health insurance if it were embodied in a plan providing services of the highest standard and fair both to the insured and to the physicians, clearly left unresolved a number of questions which would emerge with the development of the plan. In 1944, in an attempt to incorporate new ideas and clarify existing policy, the General Council of the Association again considered the principles upon which it claimed a health insurance plan should be based. In its revised policy the Council stated that "the plan must be compulsory for persons having an annual income insufficient to meet the costs of adequate medical care," and that "Health Insurance should be administered by an independent, non-political commission representative of those giving and those receiving the services."[11]

After 1944, a number of voluntary profession-sponsored medical care prepayment plans emerged and enrolled substantial numbers of contributors. Besides these plans there existed medical co-operatives which were organized by the consumers rather than the providers of medical care, and commercial insurance plans selling protection against medical care costs. The Canadian Medical Association recognized the growth of voluntary and other forms of prepayment and changed its view concerning the necessity for collective action on medical care insurance by government. The Association, although recognizing such action was necessary to protect those unable to afford medical care premiums and costs, now affirmed its belief in the principle of voluntary action, and in 1949 it amended its previous policy to incorporate this change in emphasis.[12]

On the basis of this principle the Association indicated its willingness to "cooperate in the preparation of detailed schemes which have as their object the removal of any barriers which exist between the people and the medical services they need." Nevertheless, the Association, although recognizing that health insurance is an appropriate mechanism for making medical care available to all, now claimed that this arrangement should be operated on a voluntary, rather than a collective basis, through the growth

10 / See appendix I.
11 / See appendix II. 12 / See appendix III.

of existing and new voluntary prepayment plans. This meant a radically different policy from the one which the Association had previously advocated. The profession indicated that it was still willing to co-operate in a government-sponsored programme, but that it now endorsed voluntary plans with the government simply assisting those unable to pay voluntary plan premiums.

In 1951 the president of the Association announced the formation of an association of voluntary medical care prepayment plans, to be called Trans-Canada Medical Plans, which would allow for transferability of prepaid medical care benefits between plans in different provinces.[13] This agency was to be used as the profession's answer to government-sponsored medical care insurance.

The Association continued to examine carefully its policy regarding health insurance and in 1955 provided a statement in which an attempt was made to distinguish between policy and principles, and to specify those principles "which affected (a) medical practice under any conditions, (b) medical care provided under voluntary prepayment arrangements and (c) those which should govern in the event of a government-sponsored plan."[14] This statement, which reaffirmed the principle of voluntary action, nevertheless recognized that such action could not achieve medical care coverage of the total population and would have to be buttressed by government assistance in extending health insurance to those who were unable to meet the costs of medical coverage.

In 1960 the General Council of the Canadian Medical Association again reconsidered its statement of principles and reiterated its basic beliefs.[15] This statement, although recognizing that some areas of medical services must be financed through taxation, asserts that a universal comprehensive medical care insurance programme financed through government-imposed taxes "is neither necessary nor desirable," but "that certain individuals require assistance" to prepay the costs of medical care. The mechanism through which those individuals unable to prepay these costs are determined is not specified, thus leaving unanswered the question of whether or not the Association believes in a means test with its implications of inequality. It is obvious that this statement recognizes that the government has a role to play in financing medical care, but it is equally obvious that there is a strong belief that voluntary insurance arrangements are of paramount importance in medical care insurance.

13 / *Globe and Mail,* June 19, 1951.
14 / Malcolm G. Taylor, "The Medical Profession and Health Insurance," unpublished mimeo. See appendix IV.
15 / See appendix V.

Before the next official statement on medical care insurance by the Canadian Medical Association two events occurred which seem to have reinforced the profession's negative attitude to government-administered medical care insurance. The dispute in 1962 between the government of Saskatchewan and the physicians of that province, as represented by the Saskatchewan College of Physicians and Surgeons, and the recommendations of the Royal Commission on Health Services in 1964 for a universal, comprehensive, publicly administered system of prepaid medical and other health care insurance apparently proved to the profession that their fears regarding this type of government health insurance were well founded. In fact, however, the continued existence of the strains faced by the physician in his professional role was crucial, and he reacted to them by focussing his resulting anxieties and frustrations on government proposals for health insurance. He used these proposals as a "scapegoat" on which he could vent those anxieties and frustrations. In Saskatchewan, where the proposed insurance scheme was implemented and with which he was forced to come to terms, his "scapegoating" of the government scheme continued. It will likely continue until his conditions of work change and lessen the strains he faces in his role or until a new "scapegoat" is found. That the former possibility may be emerging has been suggested earlier in the description of the increasing percentage of physicians in the province who have accepted a method of paying for their services which requires them to forward all claims for services directly to the Saskatchewan Medical Care Commission. This may indicate that the realities of medical practice under the Saskatchewan plan have tended to lessen at least some of the role strains of the physician.

However, in June 1965 the General Council of the Canadian Medical Association reasserted the principles governing the physician's relationship to a system of medical services insurance in a statement of policy which was similar to those put forward prior to both the Saskatchewan dispute and the Report of the Royal Commission on Health Services.[16]

16 / See appendix VI.

IO

THE CONTENT OF
THE IDEOLOGY OF
MEDICAL CARE

THROUGHOUT THE six statements on health and medical care insurance issued by the Canadian Medical Association between 1943 and 1965 certain major themes or propositions emerge which are clearly related to the one central anxiety facing the medical profession: the control by third parties, particularly public medical care insurance commissions or agencies, over the conditions of work of the physician. This emphasis is to be expected in official statements on medical care insurance by the profession. Other themes are also evident which are related to other types of strain in the role of the physician, but limitations of space make it impossible to analyse every strand in the medical ideology manifested in these statements. The selection of some themes rather than all of them for analysis is based upon two criteria. The first is an assessment of the closeness of their relationship to present and possible future strains in the role of the physician attributable to the impact of existing and proposed medical care insurance schemes on the social organization of medical practice, and their relationship to major societal values. The second is the frequency with which these themes or propositions occur in one form or another in the successive statements. A study of appendices I to VI will reveal that the relationship between themes or propositions, role strains, and societal values is clearest in the most frequently repeated themes.

These themes are illustrated below in selected extracts taken from the official statements. To include in this analysis every extract containing one or more of the themes would be clearly redundant since the various themes or propositions contained in the successive statements are stated with the following approximate frequencies during the period 1943–65.[1]

1 / Some difficulty was encountered in the attempt to specify the thematic content of the various statements. Unless the theme could be interpreted relatively unam-

	Frequency	*Rank*
Professional control	16	1
Freedom	13	2
Quality of medical care	12	3
Public responsibility	7	4
Privacy	5	5
Personal responsibility	4	6
Voluntary participation	4	6
Universal availability	4	6

As noted above professional control over the conditions of work is the most persistent concern of the profession evident in these periodic statements, closely followed by freedom of the physician and the individual patient, and the quality of medical care. In the statements of the Association these three themes are closely associated, that is, professional control, freedom, and quality are seen as interdependent factors in medical practice. In the following analysis, however, each of them will be discussed separately in order to specify more clearly the particular characteristics of each which reflect role strains and their link with community values. The remaining themes, public responsibility, privacy, personal responsibility, voluntary participation, and universal availability, will be discussed mainly in terms of the association of one with another, e.g., public responsibility and personal responsibility, which is evident in the statements.

The various themes which appear in the ideology of medical care receive a varying emphasis during the period 1943–1965. Using the approximate frequencies noted above the distribution appears as shown in Table 11. It is evident that in 1944 the medical profession stressed those themes which it felt were related to the issue of a government health and medical care insurance programme. By 1949, with the emergence of voluntary, physician-sponsored prepayment schemes, the profession stressed themes associated with this development such as public responsibility for those families and individuals unable to afford the cost of the premiums required for the physician-sponsored plans, and the concept of voluntary participation. By 1965, however, having experienced the Saskatchewan medical care dispute and with the recommendations of the Royal Commission on Health Services to consider as a future possibility, the profession stressed freedom and autonomy above all other conditions.

---

biguously, it was not counted. This means that others who study the statements for a count of the same themes may find different frequencies, but it is felt that these differences would not change the ranking of the themes.

TABLE 11
Frequency of Specific Themes Appearing in Periodic Statements on Health Insurance
by Canadian Medical Association, 1943–65

	1943	1944	1949	1955	1960	1965	Total
Professional control		5		4	5	2	16
Freedom		2		1	4	6	13
Quality of medical care	1	2		5	1	3	12
Public responsibility			3	3		1	7
Privacy		2		1	1	1	5
Personal responsibility			2	1		1	4
Voluntary participation			1	2		1	4
Universal availability			1		1	2	4

PROFESSIONAL CONTROL AND SELF-GOVERNMENT

The profession's concern over the effect of a health and medical care insurance programme on professional control of all matters affecting conditions of practice is evident in the following extracts.[2]

The introduction of health insurance legislation should be preceded by adequate consultation with the organized medical profession. ... (IV)

Appointments of medical personnel to the [Health Insurance] Commission and its staff should be made only with the approval of organized medicine in the respective province. (IV)

The competence and ability of any doctor is determined by professional self-government. (VI)

This insurance should cover the services of the physician in the home, office, or hospital, and ... the services of paramedical personnel working under his direction and professional services and therapeutic agents otherwise ordered by him. (VI)

Members of the medical profession, as the providers of services, have the right to determine the method of their remuneration. (V)

The amount of remuneration is a matter of negotiation between the physician and his patient or those acting on their behalf; and ... all medical service programs [should] make provision for periodic or automatic changes in remuneration to reflect changes in economic conditions. (V)

These extracts highlight a number of difficulties facing the professional association and the practising physician. If control of individual members of the medical profession is to be maintained by the professional associa-

2 / To obviate the necessity for numerous footnotes to the specific appendix from which each extract was taken, each extract will be followed by the number of the appendix of which it is a part, in parentheses.

tion it must be recognized by government and other third parties as the official spokesman of the profession. Lack of such recognition would result in individual negotiations between each physician and third parties on matters affecting the interests of the physician, with a consequent weakening of group loyalties and group structure.

Continued acceptance by governments, third parties, and individuals of the claim that a physician's competence and ability can be determined only by the professional body strengthens group loyalties and builds professional solidarity. The weakening or lack of acceptance of this principle would weaken group loyalties, and decrease the strength of formal sanctions hitherto applied by the professional body with a possible lowering of standards of service by an individual physician. Lack of support outside the profession for the principle of professional self-government and control would mean that a physician was deprived of the formal support of his peers and his association in his dealings with other professions, patients, and third parties. A physician may chafe at the controls, formal or informal, imposed on his professional behaviour by his peers since these controls produce strain and anxiety as he attempts to apply his skills in a changing medical world in which the possibility of error is increasing. Nevertheless, the benefits of organization and co-operation centred in his professional association are a protection against the vicissitudes of practice and outweigh the strains resulting from the possibility of professional sanctions.

In its efforts to control the working conditions of its members the professional body seeks to maintain its authority over other occupations and professions with which the professional person actively associates in his practice. As indicated in chapter 5, for example, the hospital is a seed bed of professionalization of paramedical skills and the practitioners of these skills are constantly striving for professional status. The physician must increasingly depend upon them for the effective discharge of his own responsibilities, and this dependence creates a situation in which these practitioners seek to compete for status and prestige with the physician.[3] To ensure that the status of the physician remains superior to that of the paramedical practitioner the medical profession makes the claim that in a health insurance scheme paramedical personnel should work under the direction of physicians. Furthermore, at least one provincial college of physicians and surgeons has suggested that the licensing of paramedical personnel should be undertaken through the college.[4]

Professional self-government and professional autonomy are two of the

3 / See p. 81.
4 / See p. 89.

rewards which society provides for the achievement of professional status. Since achievement is a recognized value in Canadian society, these and other rewards, such as status, prestige, and income, are the incentives which that society offers for achievement in professional or other areas of activity. The demand by a professional body that professional self-govern-ment and autonomy should continue to be fully recognized is itself a recognition that they are the rewards of achievement.

The fear that the system of rewards may be somehow changed and that particular rewards may be lessened is evident, for example, in the extracts concerning the right of medical practitioners to determine the method and amount of their remuneration. The profession is well aware that different methods of remuneration provide opportunities by third parties for more or less interference in the practice of medicine. Physicians in salaried posi-tions are more vulnerable to third party interference in professional mat-ters than those paid according to a fee-for-service system. The salary as a method of remuneration is one of the significant working conditions of bureaucratic organizations in which the employer has the power to control the activities of employees. The fee-for-service system of remuneration, on the other hand, is a crucial organizational element in solo practice by which the independent, solo practitioner can maintain a high degree of professional autonomy; he can control his working conditions to a far greater extent than the salaried physician holding a position in a bureau-cratic organization. This system of remuneration is thus a vital element in the maintenance of the present organizational structure of medical care with its emphasis on professional control and autonomy. Here is one of the reasons why the possibility of a change in the organization of medical care, which would require some method of paying the physician other than the fee-for-service method, arouses the physician's fears and anxieties. Furthermore, the fee method of payment is associated with a competitive society in which professional achievement is recognized by the freedom of the practitioner to charge fees within the limits imposed by his profession and the demand for professional services. The prospect of a change to some other system of remuneration generates the fear that the recognition of achievement will become less important, so that during a practitioner's career the rise in income will slow down with the result that differences in income level between different types of practitioners – such as between specialists and general practitioners – and at different stages of a practi-tioner's career will decrease. The medical profession believes that there should be no restrictions on income, other than those which it recognizes at present, and that a fee-for-service practitioner should be free to earn an income of whatever size the demand for his service generates.

FREEDOM

The emphasis on freedom in the following excerpts connects certain propositions in the ideology of medical care with one of Canada's major social values, and by so doing it tends to legitimize these ideological claims in the eyes of the community as well as the physician. At the same time it indicates certain strains which are evident in the physician's role.

Every resident of Canada is free to select his doctor and ... each doctor is free to choose his patients. (v)

Each individual physician is free to select the type and location of his practice. (v)

... every resident of Canada should have as free a choice as possible among different carriers and different plans [of prepaid medical insurance], ... and ... every physician should ... be free to participate, or not to participate, in any plan or with any carrier. (vi)

We believe that it is in every sense in the public interest that these freedoms be preserved. (vi)

The Canadian Medical Association confidently believes that the people of this nation can develop insurance programs which will preserve freedom of individual choice and action ... (vi)

By emphasizing freedom as a value in these statements, for both the consumer and the provider of medical services, the medical profession once again legitimizes its status as a free, autonomous, self-governing profession. A patient, too, should be free; free to choose his own physician, despite the fact that patients who "shop around" for what they conceive to be a suitable physician may create competition between physicians. It is not clear whether the patient who is dissatisfied with the medical care he receives should be free to seek the services of another physician, a situation which could result in invidious comparisons in addition to competition among physicians.

The emphasis on a practitioner's freedom to choose his patient, and the type and location of practice, is related to the difficulties many doctors face today in meeting the rising demand for medical services under the conditions of solo and some other forms of private practice. A solo practitioner is a private entrepreneur who invests the necessary capital to provide the facilities and personnel to equip and operate his office. The organization of this type of practice may produce difficulties in satisfying the demand for these services. Since he may be unable to meet this demand the physician must be free to curtail it by choosing his patients, particularly when some of them make what he views as excessive and unreasonable demands on his skill, time, and other resources.

The type of practice in which the physician is engaged is related to the amount of his income. Private practitioners, particularly specialists, whether in solo, group, or some other type of private practice, on the average, usually earn higher incomes than physicians in non-private practice in government. Any threat to the freedom of choice of practice, particularly if this means practice under the authority of a public agency such as a health insurance commission, arouses the anxiety of a physician, who views such working arrangements as limiting his income and his autonomy.

Freedom to determine the location of practice is related to the maldistribution of physicians. With increasing urbanization population is concentrated in urban areas and in order to meet the demand for medical care of the large urban population groups, hospitals and other medical services tend to concentrate in these areas. Physicians are attracted to these centres because of the availability of services and facilities. On the other hand, in the less heavily populated rural areas the demand for services is appreciably lower with the result that facilities and services are relatively scarce when compared with metropolitan and other urban centres. Physicians are therefore reluctant to practice in rural areas. Their fears are aroused when they assume that third parties, particularly public health insurance agencies, may act to relieve the maldistribution of physicians by restricting their freedom to locate where they wish and possibly directing some to under-serviced areas.

The anxiety and strain among physicians as a result of what they see as the possibility of limitations imposed by government controlled and administered medical care insurance on the freedoms outlined above provided the incentive for the organization of physician-sponsored medical care prepayment plans, as well as the profession's endorsement of commercial medical care insurance plans. These were the profession's answer to government plans despite the fact that they placed some limited restrictions on the physician's autonomy, particularly in the case of the physician-sponsored plans.[5] Nevertheless, the role strains which these conditions created were preferred to those much more severe strains which the profession saw resulting from physicians working for a government medical care insurance agency. The proposition that a physician should be free to participate, or not to participate, in government or any other plans leaves it up to the individual physician to decide the conditions under which he wishes to practise. The linking of this particular freedom of the physician with the freedom of the citizen to have a free choice among various plans tends to place physician and citizen in a similar situation in which they are both seen as seeking to realize the rights of

5 / See chapter 7.

free people. In this way the medical profession legitimizes these particular propositions and thereby protects the interests of its members. This aim is quite obvious in the statement of the belief that it is in the public interest that these freedoms be preserved and that Canadians can develop insurance plans that will preserve freedom of individual choice. Here the particular conditions the profession wishes to perpetuate or create, which it assumes would reduce existing and possible future role strains, are linked to freedom as a social value and thereby legitimized for the profession and the public.

QUALITY

The quality of medical care is frequently stressed in the official statements of the medical profession concerning health and medical care insurance.

The highest standards of medical care should be available to every resident of Canada. (v)

The Canadian Medical Association ... will gladly participate in the formulation of programmes designed to make high quality medical services more readily available and which respect the essential principles of medical practice. (IV)

If a system were created which undertook to pay the total cost of health services and were dependent for this on a single and therefore potentially limited source of funds, it could be obliged through lack of restraint to do one of two things.
   A   to impose restrictions on the coverage of people or of services, or
   B   to be in continual conflict with the providers of service over working conditions and remuneration.
We believe that such restrictions or conflicts would impair the quality of care, and we believe it is not in the public interest that a plan be established which cannot be readily adjusted without restriction or conflict. (VI)

... the extension of coverage to the whole population, especially on a total prepayment basis, will place a considerable strain on available personnel and may endanger the quality of the care which the public receives. (VI)

In the provision of personal health services where the usual doctor-patient relationship exists, it is the view of the Canadian Medical Association that remuneration on a basis of fee-for-services rendered promotes high quality of care. (IV)

The Canadian Medical Association favours a plan of health insurance which will secure the development and provision of the highest standards of health care ... if such a plan be fair to both the insured and to all those rendering the services. (I)

The quality of medical care depends on a number of factors, which include the supply, availability, knowledge, skill, and commitment of professionally qualified physicians, on the medical facilities at their disposal, and on the organization of their services.[6] The medical profession is well aware of this relationship, but it is also aware that in so far as the individual physician is concerned his ability to supply sufficient services to meet the increasing demand for them, the difficulties associated with maintaining an adequate level of skill and knowledge, the conflicting pressures which tend to dampen his commitment, the lack of co-ordination among and sometimes the inadequate level of facilities, and the manner in which his services are organized, particularly in private solo practice, all tend to create strains in his role. The nature of those strains related to the quality of care is evident in the foregoing excerpts. The profession reacts to them by reiterating certain basic ideological themes which it associates with general societal values.

According to the profession, high quality medical care is not readily available to all – a recognition that the demand for such care exceeds the ability of the profession to meet it. But any proposals for solving this problem, whether by government or any other agency, must, it states, be based on an acceptance of the principles of medical practice, i.e., professional autonomy and self-government. The fear that government-controlled medical care insurance agencies would interfere in the principles of practice is evident in the statement that a single source of funds, such as those raised by government through taxation mechanisms, premiums, or both, would be in conflict with physicians over working conditions and remuneration. Government financing of such an insurance scheme would necessitate a high degree of government budgetary control and would probably result in some type of quality review, as is evident at present to a limited extent in both government and voluntary medical care insurance programmes. Such a review might indicate sharp differences in the quality of care provided by physicians. These differences might very well lead to the government insurance agency seeking some arrangement whereby the quality of medical care can be improved. Such interference in the autonomy of a practitioner obviously would create severe role strains for him. The profession attempts to justify and gain support for its position in this matter by claiming that the insured, as well as the physician, would suffer restrictions in terms of the service provided by the insurance. Further justification is sought by suggesting that such interference and restrictions are not in the public interest. In other words, the profession's control over working conditions *is* in the public interest.

The profession is cognizant of the strains the physician faces as he seeks

6 / Royal Commission on Health Services, *Final Report*, vol. II, p. 1.

to meet the increasing demand for medical care. These strains would be increased if the rate of increase in this demand were to rise as a result of the introduction of a universal medical care insurance scheme. There appears to be an implicit assumption underlying the profession's aware- ness of this situation that the existing medical care system fails to meet part of the present demand. It is apparent, however, that rising demand for medical care under the present system of providing it would substan- tially increase the role strains of the physician and thereby endanger pre- vailing quality standards. To maintain and possibly improve these stan- dards in the face of a sharply rising demand would require changes in the working conditions of physicians such as noted earlier, particularly in the manner in which physicians' services are organized and delivered.

The Canadian Medical Association links high quality of medical care with the fee-for-service system of remuneration which is associated with private practice, i.e., solo, partnership, or group practice. Each of these forms of practice provides more or less opportunity for interference in the physician's role from both peers and laymen, including patients, which can create strain and thereby affect quality; in some instances, quality may be improved, in others it may be lowered. But as indicated earlier[7] quality is also affected by factors such as the supply, availability, knowledge, and skill of physicians. Since all these factors affect quality, the claim by the Canadian Medical Association that the fee-for-service system of remu- neration promotes quality of medical care is obviously too selective, if not distorted. On the other hand, knowing the concern of medical care in- surance officials, whether government or voluntary, and the general public with the quality of care provided by physicians, the Association by relating quality to the fee-for-service system of payment seeks government and community support for that system. The attempt to gain community sup- port for its ideological claims is also evident in the Association's assertion that it is in favour of a health insurance plan that will provide the highest standards of care, which is tied in with a prevailing social value in the declaration that such a plan must be fair to all.

PUBLIC RESPONSIBILITY, PRIVATE RESPONSIBILITY, VOLUNTARY PARTICIPATION AND UNIVERSAL AVAILABILITY

The belief in the principle of public responsibility is probably more noticeable in Canada than in the United States. This stems from an histori- cal reliance on government action to protect the integrity of Canadian institutions which have faced the competitive power of similar institutions

7 / See p. 56.

in the United States. In order to maintain this integrity in the face of such pressure successive Canadians have actively supported and sometimes built and controlled certain Canadian institutions. As noted in chapter 9 this historical tradition is evident in the founding of the Canadian railway system and more recently in the building of Air Canada and the Canadian Broadcasting Corporation. This is not to suggest that active government support of certain institutions is not evident also in the United States. In that country, however, the belief in the principle of public responsibility is overshadowed by the belief in the principle of private responsibility and initiative. This latter principle is evident, too, in Canada, but here it is probably less dominant than in the United States.

The ideology of medical care includes both these beliefs or themes, with public responsibility being stressed more often than private responsibility.

The Canadian Medical Association confidently believes that the people of this nation can develop insurance programmes which will preserve freedom of individual choice and action, foster personal initiative and responsibility, and while so doing make adequate insurance coverage possible for every Canadian. (VI)

The Canadian Medical Association ... having seen demonstrated the successful application of the insurance principle in the establishment of the voluntary prepaid medical care plans recommends the extension of these plans to cover all residents of Canada with financial assistance from public funds where this is required. (IV)

The Canadian Medical Association ... recommends, where it becomes evident that the voluntary medical care plans cannot achieve adequate coverage, that provincial governments collaborate in the administrative and financial task of extending health insurance to all through the medium of the voluntary prepayment plans. (IV)

The first of these statements illustrates clearly the manner in which the profession attempts to legitimize its claims and recommendations by linking them with the societal values of individual choice, personal initiative, and responsibility.

The two following statements, which associate the themes of public responsibility, voluntary participation and universal availability, are more indicative of certain difficulties which the profession faces as it seeks to extend the coverage of the physician-sponsored plans to the total population. The profession is aware that the cost of the prepayment premiums of these plans is beyond the means of substantial numbers of the population.[8] Nevertheless, it must retain some control over these plans if it is to protect the interest of the individual physician in maintaining his existing

8 / See p. 190.

practice arrangements in which, particularly in private solo practice, he is allowed a high degree of professional freedom with only limited control by his peers. To leave the total responsibility for prepaid medical care insurance in government hands would mean more control. Thus the profession seeks to expand the enrolment in the voluntary physician-sponsored plans by seeking government assistance in the form of the payment of the cost, or some part of it, of the premiums which a number of individuals and families cannot afford. Such an arrangement leaves the profession in control of the plans except for some budgetary and possibly other restrictions relating to the costs required to subsidize the plans for covering those unable to afford their premiums.

As members of Canadian society, physicians hold certain values in common with other members of society. Voluntary effort and equality are values which direct much of the activity of Canadians. It is not unexpected, therefore, that the medical profession should stress them as guiding principles in organizing medical care insurance, while at the same time specifying the necessity for government support for such a plan. But by making voluntary effort and universal availability, with its connotations of equality of access to medical services, basic elements of a plan requiring government support, the profession justifies to the public, the government, and physicians an arrangement that would lessen the possibility of interference in professional matters.

PRIVACY

Although a person's social class affects his attitude towards privacy there can be little doubt that it is a widely held value in Canadian society, particularly with respect to one's body. As we have indicated previously,[9] society accepts the fact that a physician must have access to his patient's body which is unavailable to others; he is privy also to the most intimate details of the life of his patient. The theme of privacy and confidentiality is evident in statements by the profession as illustrated in the following excerpts.

The confidential nature of the patient-doctor relationship must remain inviolate ... (IV)

Among the safeguards which should be given to the public, one of the most important is that of privacy. Payment for any insured service has to be justified by a diagnosis and often by other medical information. The relationship between patient and physician must nevertheless be kept as private as possible, and any information provided to the insurer must be used solely for the assessment of claims and must be handled consistently in a confidential manner. (VI)

9 / See p. 17.

The threat of third party intervention in the private and confidential relationship between physician and patient can be an effective weapon by which the former may prevent any type of interference in the conduct of medical practice. The medical profession is fully aware of the potential for various types of interference by third parties from past experience with the medical care insurance plans which it has itself sponsored. Although this limited interference has been accepted by the profession, despite the strains it has created in the role of the physician, the possibility of a medical care insurance scheme supported by the statutory and financial power of government raises the hazards, from the profession's point of view, of further, more restrictive interference in matters relating to conditions of practice such as fees, quality, facilities, therapy, and the organization, choice, and location of practice. Such a situation creates the potential for greatly increased strains in the physician's role. To protect itself from this possibility the profession emphasizes the private and confidential nature of the physician-patient relationship, which has value implications for other members of society.

The foregoing excerpts derived from the periodic official statements of the Canadian Medical Association during the period 1943–65 illustrate the chief characteristics of an ideology: selectivity, oversimplification, and the use of symbols. These are important links between ideology and role strain.

Faced with the incompatible or conflicting demands of his role, the physician experiences strain. Nevertheless, he must decide in a given situation on a course of action. His decision may be based on rational principles which have an obvious empirical basis, but it is the function of ideology at all times to guide his action and relieve strains.[10] For example, the anxiety created by the fear of intervention by government and other agencies in the financing of medical care has generated the medical profession's claims that the quality of patient care will be lowered, or at least endangered, if government pays the medical care bill. There is an obvious selectivity and an oversimplification in this element in the medical ideology. The quality of medical care bears no necessary relationship to the source of fee payment. Such an assertion disregards many other factors related to the quality of medical care provided by a physician.

10 / Limitations on the theory of the relationship between ideology and role strains are discussed in Francis X. Sutton *et al.*, *The American Business Creed*, Cambridge, Mass.: Harvard University Press, 1956, pp. 308–9. Sutton points out that there is no exact correspondence between particular strains and specific ideological items; a person can respond to strain in a number of other ways; "the ideology is a symbolic outlet for the emotional energy which the strain creates."

The symbolic element in the ideology of the medical profession is exemplified in statements such as those dealing with "fairness," "freedom," and "personal initiative and responsibility." These are value symbols which designate those aspects of their society which physicians wish to perpetuate and which are indeed part of the Canadian cultural heritage. Such symbolization, of course, overlooks the complexities of the society to which it refers, but since this complexity cannot be integrated into the ideology, it must be simplified to portray the society in a plausible fashion.

All established professions have shared values and expectations which are generated by ties between colleagues and provide for their practitioners "the meaning of the occupation and its place in the world."[11] In a period of change affecting the professional role, a professional association seeks to emphasize the legitimacy of its professional culture for the lay public and its own practitioners. As is evident in the foregoing statements, this attempt is made by linking certain professional ideological themes to general social values. In this process these values are purposely related to widely held images of the profession, which "may be true images," but which are "allowed to engulf or obscure contrary truth and images and so become professional fictions. These fictions help to define immediate functions; they help the professional person to relate to others in terms of some mutuality of expectancy."[12] For the practitioner the continued emphasis on the professional cultural themes generates ideological consensus; it also strengthens collegial ties, and thereby promotes professional solidarity.

11 / Harvey L. Smith, "Contingencies of Professional Differentiation," *American Journal of Sociology*, vol. 63, 1957–58, p. 412.
12 / *Ibid.*, p. 413.

I I

IDEOLOGICAL CONSENSUS

A PERSON's ideological beliefs can indicate his preference for a particular side of an argument. The beliefs used in such a situation are derived from the groups of which the person is a member, or aspires to become a member. These reference groups are used as models by the individual with different reference groups usually being used for different subjects of belief.[1] Similarity of ideological beliefs in social groups depends upon the homogeneity of social background of the members of the groups; the greater this homogeneity in social characteristics, such as occupation or profession, class, age, sex, ethnic group, and religious affiliation, the greater the intensity with which the beliefs will be held, and the higher the probability that they will be used to guide behaviour.[2] Social groups face issues some of which may require group action; the more important the issue for the group the greater the agreement among its members on the beliefs concerning the issue.[3]

To determine the degree of similarity in ideological belief in the medical profession on the issue of medical care insurance administered and financed by government would require some measurement of the factors noted above as affecting that ideological consensus. Unfortunately, no precise measures are available concerning the range of factors affecting the ideological beliefs noted in the previous chapter. Some data are available, however, on sponsorship by the medical profession of various medical care insurance plans; this reflects physicians' belief in professional control and autonomy, the most frequently reiterated theme in the successive statements on medical care insurance issued by the Canada Medical Association. Limited data are also available on the class background of physicians which can be related to this belief, plus other data on type of work, employing agency, location of practice and type of remuneration

1 / Bernard Berelson and Gary A. Steiner, *Human Behaviour: An Inventory of Scientific Findings*, New York: Harcourt, Brace and World, Inc., 1964, p. 558.
2 / *Ibid.*, p. 567.
3 / *Ibid.*, p. 568.

which deal more specifically with the characteristics of the professional group itself.

These data are derived from the 1962 Survey of Physicians in Canada referred to in previous chapters. In this Survey every physician practising or retired in Canada was asked a number of questions designed to elicit his beliefs and opinions about current plans of medical insurance and possible future developments.[4] One question sought to ascertain the physician's preference for various types of sponsorship of a medical care insurance plan, i.e., the medical profession, government, an insurance company, or some other type of sponsorship. The physician could choose any one, or any combination of types of sponsorship.

PROFESSIONAL SOLIDARITY

Table 12 indicates that of the 11,181 physicians answering this question, 62.0 per cent preferred the sponsorship of the medical profession. The occupational background of these physicians, as determined by father's occupation at the time his offspring entered university appears to make little difference to the degree of solidarity among physicians on this issue. Of these respondents 58.8 per cent had fathers with managerial, professional, or technical occupations, which fall largely in the upper occupational classes when classified according to the Blishen scale.[5] In both these groups the preference expressed was identical with that of all respondents combined; at least 62.0 per cent of them preferred the medical profession to sponsor a medical care insurance plan. A clear majority of physicians with different occupational class backgrounds also preferred this type of sponsorship, the range being from 55.7 per cent for physicians with fathers' occupations not stated to 72.2 per cent for those whose fathers were miners, quarrymen, etc. The next most preferred type of sponsorship is that of the insurance company but it is preferred by a much smaller percentage of physicians no matter what their fathers' occupational background.

If the homogeneity of the class background of individuals tends to stimulate ideological consensus within a group and the intensity with which beliefs will be held, we could expect that some significant percentage differences in preference for medical profession sponsorship would appear in Table 12 between physicians with different occupational class origins.

4 / S. Judek, *Medical Manpower in Canada*, Royal Commission on Health Services, Ottawa: Queen's Printer, 1964, p. 308.

5 / Bernard R. Blishen, "A Socio-Economic Index for Occupations in Canada," *Canadian Review of Sociology and Anthropology*, vol. 4, no. 1, 1967.

TABLE 12
Percentage Distribution for Canada of Physicians by Preferred Sponsorship of a Medical Insurance Plan by Father's Occupation, 1962 (N = 11,181)

Father's occupation at time of entering university	Preferred sponsorship of medical insurance plan									
	Medical profession	Govt.	Insurance co.	Other	Medical profession and/or govt.	Medical profession and/or insurance co.	Govt. and/or insurance co.	Medical profession, insurance co. govt.	Not stated	Total
Managerial	62.1	7.4	17.9	3.2	1.1	2.3	0.1	0.6	5.3	100.0
Professional, technical	62.0	7.7	17.0	3.4	1.8	2.2	0.2	0.6	4.9	99.8
Clerical	58.7	9.3	21.4	3.4	1.4	1.1	0.5	0.2	3.9	100.0
Sales	62.5	7.0	19.5	1.9	1.5	3.4	—	—	4.2	100.0
Service and recreation	65.4	9.2	12.5	5.4	0.8	2.1	—	—	4.6	100.0
Transportation, communication	59.3	9.2	17.4	3.7	4.3	2.1	—	0.9	3.1	100.0
Farmers and farm workers	64.3	7.4	15.8	2.5	1.5	2.8	0.5	0.5	4.7	100.0
Loggers, related workers	68.6	5.9	11.8	2.0	—	5.9	—	—	5.9	100.0
Fishermen, trappers, hunters	61.5	15.4	7.7	—	—	—	—	—	15.4	100.0
Miners, quarrymen, etc.	72.2	8.3	16.7	2.8	—	—	—	—	—	100.0
Craftsmen, productive process	62.5	8.3	18.1	2.8	1.6	2.1	—	0.3	4.3	100.0
Labourers	61.5	6.0	22.5	1.5	3.5	2.0	—	0.5	2.5	100.0
Not stated	55.7	10.9	13.1	3.7	2.7	3.7	0.5	0.5	9.2	100.0
Total	62.0	7.8	17.4	3.1	1.6	2.4	0.2	0.5	4.9	99.9

SOURCE: Royal Commission on Health Services, Survey of Physicians in Canada, 1962.

But since an overwhelming proportion in each class preferred medical profession sponsorship, we can assume that differences in class of origin among members of the medical profession have little effect in generating consensus around this issue.

The continuing solidarity of the profession on the issue of the sponsorship of medical care insurance is also evident in Table 13. Regardless of the year they were first licensed to practise, the majority of the physicians in this Survey preferred the sponsorship of the medical profession, and again the next most preferred type of sponsorship is that by the insurance company.

Similarly, as shown in Table 14, regardless of the type of work in which the physicians were engaged at the time of the Survey professional solidarity on this issue is evident. Nevertheless, it is interesting to note the difference between general practitioners and specialists with regard to the type of sponsorship which each group prefers for a medical insurance plan. The general practitioners show 68.6 per cent preferring medical profession sponsorship as against 57.7 of specialists. A slightly higher percentage of specialists than general practitioners prefer government or insurance company sponsorship.

The same general pattern emerges from the data in Table 15, which shows a high degree of solidarity on the issue regardless of the agency or context in which the physician is employed. Here, however, there are some interesting differences between physicians practising under different arrangements. Of those in a bureaucratic type of practice such as a government agency, or an insurance company 56.5 per cent prefer the sponsorship of the profession compared with 61.5 in solo practice, 70.6 per cent in group practice, and 71.8 per cent in partnership practice. One is tempted to make the assumption on the basis of these differences in the percentages between bureaucratic and other forms of practice that the degree of solidarity within the medical profession on this issue of the sponsorship of a medical insurance plan depends to some extent on the context of practice. This assumption also invites acceptance in view of the fact that 14.6 per cent of physicians employed by a bureaucracy prefer government, i.e., bureaucratic, sponsorship, almost three times the percentage preferring this form of sponsorship who were self-employed and between three and four times the percentage of those in partnership or group practice. However, the percentage favouring professional sponsorship among solo practitioners is only 4.8 percentage points more than among physicians employed by a bureaucracy. For partnership and group practitioners, on the other hand, the difference is 15.3 and 14.1 percentage

TABLE 13

Percentage Distribution of Physicians by Preferred Sponsorship of a Medical Insurance Plan by Year First Licensed to Practise in Canada, 1962 (N = 11,181)

Year first licensed to practise	Preferred sponsorship of medical insurance plan									
	Medical profession	Govt.	Insurance co.	Other	Medical profession and/or govt.	Medical profession and/or insurance co.	Govt. and/or insurance co.	Medical profession, Insurance co., govt.	Not stated	Total
Before 1923	62.1	9.3	12.9	1.8	1.8	3.2	0.5	0.2	8.4	100.2
1923–27	62.3	9.6	13.6	1.6	2.3	2.8	—	0.7	7.0	99.9
1928–32	65.8	6.8	13.4	2.7	1.6	2.3	0.2	0.5	6.6	99.9
1933–37	68.8	6.5	12.2	2.9	2.2	2.4	—	0.1	4.7	99.8
1938–42	62.7	5.8	16.5	4.0	1.8	2.8	0.5	1.2	4.7	100.0
1943–47	62.4	5.2	19.3	3.2	1.2	2.6	0.3	0.9	4.8	99.9
1948–52	59.2	7.7	19.7	3.6	1.8	2.7	0.2	0.7	4.4	100.0
1953–57	62.0	7.2	19.1	3.3	1.3	1.9	0.1	0.5	4.5	99.9
1958 and later	63.1	9.7	16.5	2.9	1.4	1.9	—	0.2	4.3	100.0
Not given	53.1	12.8	19.8	3.1	2.8	2.3	0.8	—	5.4	100.1
Total	62.0	7.8	17.4	3.1	1.6	2.4	0.2	0.5	4.9	99.9

SOURCE: Royal Commission on Health Services, Survey of Physicians in Canada, 1962.

TABLE 14

Percentage Distribution for Canada of Physicians by Preferred Sponsorship of Medical Insurance Plan by Type of Work in which Now Engaged, 1962 (N = 11,181)

Preferred sponsorship of medical insurance plan

Type of work	Medical profession	Govt.	Insurance co.	Other	Medical profession and/or govt.	Medical profession and/or insurance co.	Govt. and/or insurance co.	Medical profession, govt., insurance co.	Not stated	Total
General practitioners*	68.6	5.2	14.6	2.3	1.4	2.7	0.2	0.4	4.5	99.9
Specialists†	57.7	9.0	19.7	3.5	1.9	2.3	0.2	0.6	5.1	100.0
Other‡	60.2	10.5	16.4	4.0	1.3	1.6	0.3	0.3	5.3	99.9
Total	62.0	7.8	17.4	3.1	1.6	2.4	0.2	0.5	4.9	99.9

*"General practioners" include: general private practice; hospital staff, general practice; general practice, not private hospital.

†"Specialists" include: specialist, private practice; consultant, private practice; hospital staff specialist; research; teaching; public health; industrial medicine; specialist, not private hospital; consultant, not private hospital.

‡"Other" includes: junior intern; senior intern; resident fellow; hospital staff, other; hospital staff, medical director; Medical assessment; non-hospital, medical director; other.

SOURCE: Royal Commission on Health Services, Survey of Physicians in Canada, 1962.

points respectively, when compared with bureaucratic practitioners. Perhaps more solo than partnership or group practitioners are disillusioned with the prevailing controls exerted by existing physician-sponsored medical insurance plans. Indeed, 20.8 per cent of solo practitioners prefer the sponsorship of commercial insurance companies, compared with 12.9 per cent of those in partnership practice, 13.3 per cent in group practice, and 15.4 per cent in bureaucratic practice. The 15.4 per cent employed by a bureaucracy who prefer this form of sponsorship may seem an anomalous finding, but it should be pointed out that of the 3,417 physicians indicated in Table 15 as employed by a bureaucracy only about one-third were employed by government, where favourable attitudes towards government sponsorship would prevail, and the remainder were employed by universities, hospitals, industry, voluntary agencies, pharmaceutical companies, life insurance companies, and prepaid medical care plans organizations in which favourable attitudes towards insurance company sponsorship would be more likely to prevail.

A similar pattern of solidarity, reflecting substantial agreement in beliefs, is indicated in Table 16 which shows that, regardless of the size of the community in which the physicians practised, between 60 and 67 per cent preferred the sponsorship of the medical profession. Table 17 indicates that although the form in which the physician is remunerated has some bearing on the solidarity of the profession on the issue of sponsorship, the great majority prefer professional sponsorship regardless of their type of remuneration.

These data, which reflect the solidarity of the medical profession on the issue of the sponsorship of medical care insurance, provide some indication of the effect of membership in the professional group on beliefs concerning the sponsorship of a medical care insurance plan. As noted earlier, the sponsorship of such a plan has serious implications for the professional control and autonomy of medicine. These are the two most salient issues facing medicine today and the more salient an issue is to the members of a group the greater will be their agreement on group beliefs.[6] Evidence to support this proposition emerges from these tables.

Despite the many strains and pressures facing a medical practitioner, the medical ideology provides him with enough support for him to carry out his professional responsibilities. The nature of that ideology has been illustrated in the preceding pages. A physician accepts it not only because of the support it provides, but also because of certain other factors. For a physician the present organization and content of medical education, the organization of the various forms of practice and hospital activities, the

6 / Berelson and Steiner, *Human Behaviour*, p. 568.

TABLE 15
Percentage Distribution for Canada of Physicians by Preferred Sponsorship of Medical Insurance Plan by Employing Agency, 1962 (N = 11,181)

Employing agency	Preferred sponsorship of medical insurance plan									
	Medical profession	Govt.	Insurance co.	Other	Medical profession and/or govt.	Medical profession and/or insurance co.	Govt. and/or insurance co.	Medical profession, govt., insurance co.	Not stated	Total
Self	61.3	5.1	20.8	2.5	1.6	2.9	0.2	0.6	4.9	99.9
Partnership	71.8	3.7	12.9	2.7	1.4	2.3	0.2	0.5	4.5	100.0
Group	70.6	3.7	13.3	2.3	1.5	3.3	0.1	0.6	4.7	100.1
Bureaucracy*	56.5	14.6	15.4	4.4	1.8	1.3	0.2	0.4	5.2	99.8
Other†	57.1	13.1	16.1	4.2	2.4	1.8	0.6	—	4.8	100.1
Total	62.0	7.8	17.4	3.1	1.6	2.4	0.2	0.5	4.9	99.9

*Bureaucracy includes: hospitals; Department of National Health and Welfare; Department of Veterans Affairs; Canadian Pension Commission; regular armed forces; Defence Research Board; Department of National Defence; Department of Justice; other federal departments, boards, agencies; provincial departments of health; provincial hospital insurance administrations; provincial departments of education; workmen's compensation boards; other provincial departments, boards, agencies; counties or municipalities; universities or colleges; industry; Medical Research Council; voluntary agencies; pharmaceutical companies; life insurance companies; prepaid medical care and hospital plans.

†"Other" includes: other, not given.

SOURCE: Royal Commission on Health Services, Survey of Physicians in Canada, 1962.

TABLE 16
Percentage Distribution for Canada of Physicians by Preferred Sponsorship of Medical Insurance Plan by Location of Major Work in which Now Engaged, 1962 (N = 11,181)

Location	Preferred sponsorship of medical insurance plan								
	Medical profession	Govt.	Insurance co.	Other	Medical profession and/or govt.	Medical profession and/or insurance co.	Govt. and/or insurance co.	Medical profession, govt., insurance co.	Not stated	Total
Under 10,000 population	66.9	7.4	14.0	2.7	1.7	2.2	—	0.3	4.7	99.9
10–49,000	62.7	6.6	17.5	3.5	1.6	2.4	0.6	0.8	4.4	100.1
50–99,000	62.6	7.4	17.8	2.5	2.1	3.0	0.2	0.4	4.1	100.1
100,000 and over	60.5	8.2	18.2	3.3	1.6	2.4	0.2	0.5	5.1	100.0
Not stated	52.3	13.6	18.2	2.3	2.3	—	—	2.3	9.1	100.1
Total	62.0	7.8	17.4	3.1	1.6	2.4	0.2	0.5	4.9	99.9

SOURCE: Royal Commission on Health Services, Survey of Physicians in Canada, 1962.

TABLE 17

Percentage Distribution for Canada of Physicians by Preferred Sponsorship of Medical Insurance Plan by Type of Remuneration, 1962 (N = 11,181)

Type of remuneration	Preferred sponsorship of medical insurance plan								
	Medical profession	Govt.	Insurance co.	Other	Medical profession and/or govt.	Medical profession and/or insurance co.	Govt. and/or insurance co.	Medical profession, govt., insurance co.	Not stated	Total
Fees	64.6	4.5	18.4	2.6	1.5	2.8	0.2	0.6	4.8	100.0
Salary	57.9	14.4	14.7	4.4	1.8	1.5	0.2	0.3	4.8	100.0
Other	50.7	14.7	21.2	3.6	2.0	2.6	0.3	0.7	4.2	100.0
Total	62.2	7.7	17.4	3.2	1.6	2.4	0.2	0.5	4.8	100.0

SOURCE: Royal Commission on Health Services, Survey of Physicians in Canada, 1962.

degree of control exercised by colleagues and the organized profession, and his relationship with third parties, all of which impose severe strains and create anxiety, are preferred to a different medical care system. Under the present system, many physicians have achieved success or recognition, change may require new professional roles or changes in existing roles and generate new competition. The physician is emotionally committed to a career under the existing system, and from it he derives many of life's satisfactions. His emotional commitment may be such that change in existing status and prestige arrangements in the professional culture will create a threat to his personality and emotional stability. There is thus a built-in resistance to change within the profession particularly when the impetus for change comes from outside with the possibility of outside control of professional activities.

IDEOLOGY AND CHANGE

The strength of the prevailing medical ideology may prove a serious obstacle to change in the organization of medical care. Any assessment of the possibilities of such change must take into consideration the range and intensity of the pressures facing the physician today, and the degree to which he is supported by the medical ideology as he seeks to practise in the face of these pressures.

As the aspiring physician goes through medical school he is exposed to a curriculum which is slow to change despite the rapid expansion of the boundaries of knowledge. The institutional resistance to the curriculum changes that new discoveries require means that the neophyte physician to some extent is unprepared to apply the latest knowledge and techniques as he enters practice. As he becomes established in practice and attempts to meet the increasing demands for his services, the time at his disposal to attempt to close the gap between what is known and what he knows will diminish, and the gap will grow wider. In part, the increase in the demand for medical care stems from increasing per capita income which is higher than at any time in our history. Paradoxically this increase in incomes has occurred in an era when the demand for government financing of medical care has culminated in the introduction of medical care plans wholly or partly financed by most provincial governments. Furthermore, a physician must provide his services to a clientele more highly educated, more urbanized and more geographically mobile than at any time in the past; a clientele with an increasing medical sophistication and more critical of the care he provides and demanding the latest diagnostic procedures and forms of therapy.

Despite the advances in knowledge in this era of rapid social and economic change, medical education has made the physician well aware that in some areas of medicine relatively little knowledge is available, and that a large measure of uncertainty is involved in some forms of therapy. He must, nevertheless, assume the heavy responsibility for the life or death of his patients and somehow cope with the knowledge that there may be a gap between his professional efforts and their outcome. He will be aware of the growing power of medicine not only to relieve suffering, but also to increase it if new knowledge and techniques are improperly applied. Thus, he will face the psychological pressures stemming from a realization that he must somehow cope with situations in which the patient may suffer because of his acts of omission or his acts of commission. But, under a fee-for-service system of remuneration, this same physician must treat a number of patients sufficient to maintain a standard of living required of a professional person and indicative of his relative degree of success. The optimum number of patients in terms of adequate quality standards varies with the skill and experience of the practitioner, but it is obvious that quality of medical care is likely to suffer if income becomes of paramount importance to a physician, and yet this same physician must cope with the social pressures to provide evidence of his professional success in those things which money can buy. The maintenance of the quality of care may also be difficult under the traditional organizational arrangements of practice which tend to isolate the practitioner from his colleagues. In other forms of practice, quality may be better assured, but when these are forms of bureaucratic practice there may be employer demands of one sort or another that can limit the independence and professional autonomy of the practitioner.

The growing complexity of the modern general hospital can impose serious strains on a physician, whose professional advancement and economic standing may depend on his use of its services and facilities. This complexity has created a division between medical and administrative functions within the hospital, and as a result the physician may find that his professional judgments sometimes conflict with the administrative demands of the institution. He may find that if he wishes to use its facilities he must conform to administrative regulations that limit his professional autonomy. He will find, too, that the degree of colleague control, with its insistence on professional standards, may limit his sphere of competence. The range and complexity of paramedical personnel applying their skills in the hospital will pose problems for him of their appropriate use and co-ordination. Furthermore, the hospital's paramedical personnel will not only compete amongst themselves for status and prestige, but in their drive for professionalization also with the physician to whom they are responsible.

A physician may find that the demands of his professional association in terms of licensing and professional standards limit his range of activities. Furthermore, in times of social change during which the association seeks to protect the interests of the profession, the physician member may be placed under severe pressure to conform to traditional attitudes and beliefs that are part of the professional ideology.

The growth of third party medical care insurance mechanisms creates the possibility of restrictions on the independence and autonomy of the physician. The existing third party arrangements for the control of over-servicing, of fees, of quality through colleague scrutiny of particular cases, all tend to limit a physician's autonomy. The growth of government medical care insurance schemes creates an even greater potential threat of control since the expenditure of government funds for this purpose must be accounted for in the legislature with opposition parties attempting to take political advantage of any hint of waste or inefficiency. As so many physicians today correctly perceive, government budgetary control of funds required for the payment of physicians' services could lead to other types of control. Such a possibility places an increased responsibility on the profession to see that the services it provides are rationally organized and effectively applied in terms of the highest possible standards of medical care. Without the assurance that services are provided in this fashion, governments will be compelled to apply some form of control.

To accuse the medical profession of selfishness in attempting to protect its interests in the face of changes demanded by persons and groups outside the profession, or to accuse it of ignorance of the effects of social change on the organization and content of medical care is to over-simplify the nature of the difficulties facing the medical profession today. Reluctant though he may seem to accept professional change, the physician is facing a problem which is shared with other professions whose central feature is service to others. All such professions attempt to maintain control over their conditions of work as they interact with outsiders.

The future autonomy and independence of the medical profession will depend upon the manner in which its members react to the many pressures they face in a rapidly changing world. The pace of change in the social order is now placing and will continue to place heavy pressures for change on the medical care system, and particularly on that part in the system which comprises the prevailing arrangements for the delivery of medical care. This part we have termed the organization of practice, and here the medical profession has resisted structural innovation. The "freezing" of the structure of the delivery system in spite of pressures for change has resulted in severe strains for the physician. He is greatly dependent upon an ideology, with all its inevitable distortions of reality, to help to resolve the emotional conflicts, the insecurity and doubts generated by the strains he feels in the performance of his role. But this dependence can only serve to intensify institutional resistance to change and thereby create more intense strains in the future.

APPENDIX I

Statement by Canadian Medical Association
on Health Insurance, 1943

WHEREAS the objects of the Canadian Medical Association are:
1 The promotion of health and the prevention of disease;
2 The improvement of health services;
3 The performance of such other lawful things as are incidental or condu-
cive to the welfare of the public;

WHEREAS the Canadian Medical Association is keenly conscious of the desira-
bility of providing adequate health services to all the people of Canada;

WHEREAS the Canadian Medical Association has for many years been studying
plans for the securing of such health services;

THEREFORE be it resolved that:
1 The Canadian Medical Association approves the adoption of the principle
of health insurance;
2 The Canadian Medical Association favours a plan of health insurance
which will secure the development and provision of the highest standard
of health services, preventive and curative, if such plan be fair both to the
insured and to all those rendering the services.

APPENDIX II

Principles Relating to Health Insurance
Approved by the General Council of
The Canadian Medical Association, 1944

1 The Canadian Medical Association approves the adoption of the principle of contributory Health Insurance, and favours a plan which will secure the development and provision of the highest standards of health services, preventive and curative, provided the plan be fair both to the insured and to all those rendering the services.

2 Inasmuch as the health of the people depends to a great extent upon environmental conditions under which they live and work, upon security against fear and want, upon adequate nutrition, upon educational facilities, and upon the opportunities for exercise and leisure, the improvement and extension of measures to satisfy these needs should precede or accompany any future organization of medical service. Failure to provide these measures will seriously jeopardize the success of any Health Insurance plan.

3 It is not in the national interest that the State convert the whole medical profession into a salaried service.

4 It is not in the patient's interest that the State invade the professional aspects of the patient-doctor relationship. Subject to geographical and ethical restrictions this relationship includes free choice of doctor by patient and free choice of patient by doctor; it implies also maintenance of the confidential nature of medical practice.

5 While leaving to each province the decision as to persons to be included, the plan must be compulsory for persons having an annual income insufficient to meet the costs of adequate medical care.

6 The dependents of insured persons should be included in the health benefits.

7 Medical care for resident and transient indigents should be provided under the plan, the Government to pay the premiums.

8 Health benefits should be organized as follows:
  A Every regularly qualified, duly licensed medical practitioner, in good standing in the province, should be eligible to practise under the plan.
  B The benefits conferred should be such as to provide for the prevention

of disease and for the application of all necessary and adequate diagnostic and curative procedures and treatment. Specialist and consultant medical services should be available.

C The following additional services should be available through the medical practitioner:

1 Nursing service;

2 Hospital care;

3 Auxiliary services, usually in hospital;

4 Pharmaceutical service, subject to regulation.

D Dental service.

9 Cash benefits, if provided, should not be taken from the Health Insurance fund.

10 Health Insurance should be administered by an independent non-political Commission representative of those giving and those receiving the services. Matters of professional detail should be administered by committees representative of the professional groups concerned.

11 Under Health Insurance the Chief Executive Officer to the Commission and the Regional Executive Officers should be physicians appointed by the Commission from a list submitted by organized medicine in the province.

12 Each province should be served by an adequate Department of Public Health, organized on the basis of the practising physician taking an active part in the prevention of disease.

13 The granting of a license to practise medicine was designed primarily to protect the public. Therefore it is in the interests of the patient that all who desire licensure to practise a healing art should be required to conform to a uniformly high standard of preliminary education and of training in the recognized basic sciences as well as to furnish proof of adequate preparation in the clinical and technical subjects.

14 The method, or methods, of remuneration of the medical practitioners and the rate thereof, should be as agreed upon by the medical profession and the Commission of the province.

15 Every effort should be made to maintain health services at the highest possible level. This requires:

A Adequate facilities for clinical teaching in the medical colleges and hospitals;

B Post-graduate training of all medical practitioners at frequent intervals;

C Necessary facilities for and support of research.

16 The principle of insured persons being required to contribute to the insurance fund is strongly endorsed.

17 Any Health Insurance plan should be studied and approved actuarially before adoption and thereafter at periodic intervals.

18 In the provision of health services, cognizance should be taken of the fact that well over a third of Canadian doctors are now in the Armed Forces. If Health Insurance should be implemented in any province before demobilization, the interests of the medical officers in the Services should be fully protected.

APPENDIX III

Statement of Policy
Adopted by the General Council of the
Canadian Medical Association, 1949

1 The Canadian Medical Association, recognizing that health is an important element in human happiness, reaffirms its willingness in the public interest to consider any proposals, official or unofficial, which are genuinely aimed at the improvement of the health of the people.

2 Among the factors essential to the people's health are adequate nutrition, good housing and environmental conditions generally, facilities for education, exercise and leisure; and not least, wise and sensible conduct of the individual and his acceptance of personal responsibility.

3 It is recognized and accepted that the community's responsibility in the field of health includes responsibility not only for a high level of environmental conditions and an efficient preventive service, but a responsibility for ensuring that adequate medical facilities are available to every member of the community, whether or not he can afford the full cost.

4 Accordingly, the Canadian Medical Association will gladly co-operate in the preparation of detailed schemes which have as their object the removal of any barriers which exist between the people and the medical services they need and which respect the essential principles of the profession.

5 The Canadian Medical Association hopes that the provincial surveys now being conducted will provide information likely to be of value in the elaboration of detailed schemes.

6 The Canadian Medical Association, having approved the adoption of the principle of health insurance, and having seen demonstrated the practical application of this principle in the establishment of voluntary prepaid medical care plans, now proposes:

A The establishment and/or extension of these Plans to cover Canada.

B The right of every Canadian citizen to insure under these plans.

C The provision by the State of the Health Insurance premium, in whole or in part, for those persons who are adjudged to be unable to provide these premiums for themselves.

7 Additional services should come into existence by stages, the first and most urgent stage being the meeting of the costs of hospitalization for every citizen of Canada. The basic part of the cost should be met by individual contribution, the responsible governmental body bearing, in whole or in part, the cost for those persons who are unable to provide the contribution for themselves.

APPENDIX IV

The Canadian Medical Association
Statement of Policies and Principles
on Health Insurance in Canada, 1955

On the Question of Health Insurance the Canadian Medical Association:

1 Strives for the best medical care for all the people of Canada and reaffirms its long established policy of giving consideration to and co-operating in proposals, official or unofficial, that are in the public interest and genuinely aimed at the improvement of the health of the people.

2 Will gladly participate in the formulation of programmes designed to make high quality medical services more readily available and which respect the essential principles of medical practice.

3 Approves of the adoption of the principle of contributory health insurance and favours a plan or plans which will assure the development and provision of the highest standards of health service, preventive, curative and rehabilitative, provided the plan be fair both to the insured and all those rendering the services.

4 Having seen demonstrated the successful application of the insurance principle in the establishment of the voluntary prepaid medical care plans recommends the extension of these plans to cover all residents of Canada, with financial assistance from public funds where this is required.

5 Recommends, where it becomes evident that the voluntary medical care plans cannot achieve adequate coverage, that provincial governments collaborate in the administrative and financial task of extending health insurance to all through the medium of the voluntary prepayment plans.

To Maintain Consistent Progress in Health Care:

6 Health is a state of complete physical, mental and social well-being and not merely the absence of disease. Among the factors essential to the achievement of good health are adequate nutrition, good housing and healthful environmental conditions generally; facilities for education, exercise and leisure; and not least, wise and sensible conduct of the individual and his acceptance of personal responsibility for maintenance of health.

7 Each province should be adequately served by a well-organized Depart-

ment of Public Health providing personal preventive services wherever possible through the practising physician.

8 The community's responsibility for health includes not only maintenance of a high level of environmental conditions and the provision of an efficient preventive service, but assurance that adequate medical facilities and services are available to every member of the community whether or not he can afford the full cost.

9 The confidential nature of the patient-doctor relationship must remain inviolate. The patient must have freedom of choice of doctor, and the doctor free acceptance of patient except in emergency or on humanitarian grounds.

10 The granting of a license to practise medicine was designed primarily to protect the public. Therefore it is in the interest of the patient that all who desire licensure to practise a healing art should be required to conform to a uniformly high standard of preliminary education and of training in the recognized basic sciences, as well as to furnish proof of adequate preparation in the clinical and technical subjects.

11 Standards of medical services should be maintained at the highest possible level through:
   A adequate facilities for clinical teaching in the medical colleges and hospitals
   B postgraduate training for all medical practitioners at frequent intervals
   C expanded programmes of medical research.

To Assure Economy and Efficiency in the Provision of Services:

12 Hospitals, health departments, and all other health agencies should coordinate their activities so as to provide their services more effectively and economically.

13 Hospitals should be located, and their facilities and size determined on a planned, regionalized basis to assure the availability of hospitals where they are needed, the provision of technical assistance to smaller hospitals by the larger, and the ready transfer of patients as required.

14 An adequate system of institutional facilities and services requires the balanced development of diagnostic facilities, active treatment general hospitals, rehabilitation centres, chronic care facilities (including mental and tuberculosis hospitals) and home care programmes.

15 Lay and professional organizations and government health agencies should participate in community, provincial and federal health planning activities.

In the Application of the Insurance Method to Payment for Medical Services:

16 The opportunity of insuring through a prepayment medical care plan should be available to every Canadian, including dependents.

17 Benefits of a health insurance plan should include preventive, diagnostic, treatment and rehabilitation services, and the services of specialists and consultants should be available as required.

18 The methods of remuneration of medical practitioners and the rates thereof should be as agreed upon by the representative bodies of the profession and the insuring agency. In the provision of personal health services where the usual doctor-patient relationship exists, it is the view of The Canadian Medical Association that remuneration on a basis of fee for services rendered promotes high quality of medical care.

19 The provision of medical services under any plan of health insurance should be undertaken only by qualified and licensed physicians.

In the Event of Government Participation in the Universal Extension of Health Insurance to All Citizens:

20 The introduction of health insurance legislation should be preceded by adequate consultation with the organized medical profession and other groups affected.

21 Health insurance should be administered by an independent, non-political commission representative of those providing and those receiving the services. Matters of professional detail should be determined by committees of the professional groups concerned.

22 Appointments of medical personnel to the Commission and its staff should be made only with the approval of organized medicine in the respective province.

23 The various services should be introduced as benefits by stages, careful planning being given to the order in which each is introduced.

24 Cash sickness benefits, if provided, and the health services benefits should be administered from separate funds.

APPENDIX V

The Canadian Medical Association
Statement on Medical Services Insurance, 1960

The Canadian Medical Association believes that:

The highest standard of medical services should be available to every resident of Canada.

Insurance to prepay the costs of medical services should be available to all regardless of age, state of health or financial status.

Certain individuals require assistance to pay medical services insurance costs.

The efforts of organized medicine, governments and all other interested bodies should be co-ordinated towards these ends.

While there are certain aspects of medical services in which tax-supported programs are necessary, a tax-supported comprehensive program, compulsory for all, is neither necessary nor desirable.

The Canadian Medical Association will support any program of medical services insurance which adheres to the following principles:

1 That all persons rendering services are legally qualified physicians and surgeons.

2 That every resident of Canada is free to select his doctor and that each doctor is free to choose his patients.

3 That the competence and ability of any doctor is determined only by professional self-government.

4 That within his competence, each physician has the privilege to treat his patients in and out of hospital.

5 That each individual physician is free to select the type and location of his practice.

6 That each patient has the right to have all information pertaining to his medical condition kept confidential except where the public interest is paramount.

7 That the duty of the physician to his individual patient takes precedence over his obligations to any medical services insurance programs.

8 That every resident of Canada, whether a recipient or provider of services, has the right of recourse to the courts in all disputes.

9 That medical services insurance programs do not in any way preclude the private practice of medicine.

10 That medical research, undergraduate and post graduate teaching are not inhibited by any medical services insurance program.

11 That the administration and finances of medical services insurance programs are completely separate from other programs, and that any board, commission or agency set up to administer any medical services insurance program has fiscal authority and autonomy.

12 That the composite opinion of the appropriate body of the medical profession is considered and the medical profession adequately represented on any board, commission or agency set up to plan, to establish policy or to direct administration for any medical services insurance program.

13 That members of the medical profession, as the providers of medical services, have the right to determine the method of their remuneration.

14 That the amount of remuneration is a matter for negotiation between the physician and his patient, or those acting on their behalf; and that all medical services programs make provision for periodic or automatic changes in remuneration to reflect changes in economic conditions.

APPENDIX VI

The Canadian Medical Association
Statement of Policy on
Medical Services Insurance, 1965

THE NEED FOR INSURANCE

The Canadian Medical Association believes that it is in the public interest that medical services insurance be available and accessible to all Canadians.

The need for such insurance arises out of the increasing complexity and effectiveness of medical care, and the growing demand for medical services.

This insurance should cover the services of the physician in home, office, or hospital, and also, under separate accounting, the services of paramedical personnel working under his direction and professional services and therapeutic agents otherwise ordered by him.

PERSONNEL

Canada will continue to experience a shortage of physicians and of associated health personnel for at least the next generation. It will not therefore be possible to envisage unlimited availability of medical and paramedical services in the foreseeable future.

The mere provision of insurance will not of itself solve the problem of personnel, or ensure the availability of their services. In fact, the extension of coverage to the whole population, especially on a total-prepayment basis, will place a considerable strain on available personnel and may endanger the quality of the care which the public receives.

THE DANGERS OF RESTRICTIONS AND CONFLICTS

If a system were created which undertook to pay the total cost of health services, and were dependent for this on a single and therefore potentially limited source of funds, it could be obliged through lack of restraint to do one of two things:

A to impose restrictions on the coverage of people or of services,
   or
B to be in continual conflict with the providers of service over working conditions and remuneration.

We believe that such restrictions or conflicts would impair the quality of care, and we believe that it is not in the public interest that a plan be established which cannot be readily adjusted without restriction or conflict.

FLEXIBILITY AND PROGRESS

We therefore believe that alternative types of insurance, those which offer total prepayment and those which involve various forms of patient participation, must be maintained.

Time may bring into sharper relief the differences in value to the insured between various types of insurance, as well as the distinction between insurance against catastrophic costs and budgeting and prepaying of other health expenditures.

Each type of insurance has advantages and disadvantages; and medical services insurance is not the only economic protection which society requires. It would be most unfortunate if a well-meaning decision today deprived the Canadian people of choice and progress in the future.

FREEDOM

The Canadian Medical Association believes that every resident of Canada should have as free a choice as possible among different carriers and different plans, as well as a free choice of physicians; and that every physician should have free choice of patient except where humane considerations dictate the contrary, and be free to participate, or not to participate, in any plan or with any carrier.

There must be no discrimination by any insurance plan against the non-participating physician, or against the subscriber who consults him. The subscriber who consults a non-participating physician must not be obliged to relinquish any benefits for which he has directly or indirectly paid, and clear provision for his indemnification must be assured.

We believe that it is in every sense in the public interest that these freedoms be preserved. If the insurance plans devised are satisfactory to all concerned, both receivers and providers of service, then private arrangements will be relatively rare. If, on the other hand, a plan is for any reason unsatisfactory, the freedom to conclude private arrangements will be an alternative to conflict and an incentive towards improvement of the plan.

ADMINISTRATION

We believe that it is in every sense in the public interest that the administrative structures of medical services insurance programs be non-political in nature; that the medical profession be satisfactorily represented therein; and that the medical profession be fully consulted at all stages of planning and preparation.

THE ROLE OF GOVERNMENT

The development of medical services insurance is the responsibility of the provinces, and financial contributions by the federal government should not interfere with the self-determination of the provinces.

We believe that it should be the responsibility of provincial governments:

A to ensure that adequate insurance coverages with appropriate safeguards for the public, are available and accessible to every resident; and

B to provide, preferably as fixed-dollar subsidies, enough financial assistance to persons in need to enable them to purchase insurance – using the annual income-tax declaration as the basic criterion.

We believe that through co-operation between governments, insurance agencies, the public, and the medical profession, voluntary insurance can in fact be made accessible to every resident of Canada.

THE PROTECTION OF THE PUBLIC

Among the safeguards which should be given to the public, one of the most important is that of privacy. Payment for any insured service has to be justified by a diagnosis and often by other medical information. The relationship between patient and physician must nevertheless be kept as private as possible, and any information provided to the insurer must be used solely for the assessment of claims and must be handled consistently in a confidential manner.

Insurance should be offered on a universally available, guaranteed renewable basis without penalty, and provision must be made for portability and the continuation of coverage despite unemployment, illness or the death of the wage-earner.

Above all, it is in the public interest that the quality of care be maintained and enhanced. The best possible conditions of medical practice must be assured, and the fullest possible support must be given to medical and paramedical education and research.

In particular, it is a fundamental necessity that effective measures be taken to increase the output of personnel and to improve the availability of their services.

CONCLUSION

The Canadian Medical Association confidently believes that the people of this nation can develop insurance programs which will preserve freedom of individual choice and action, foster personal initiative and responsibility, and while so doing make adequate insurance coverage possible for every Canadian.

BIBLIOGRAPHY

BOOKS

Badgley, Robin F., and Samuel Wolfe, *Doctors' Strike*, Toronto: Macmillan Co., 1967.

Barber, Bernard, *Science and the Social Order*, Glencoe, Ill.: The Free Press, 1952.

Becker, Howard S., *et al.*, *Boys in White*, Chicago: University of Chicago Press, 1961.

Berelson, Bernard, and Gary A. Steiner, *Human Behaviour: An Inventory of Scientific Findings*, New York: Harcourt, Brace and World, Inc., 1964.

Berry, Charles H., *Voluntary Medical Insurance and Prepayment*, Royal Commission on Health Services, Ottawa: Queen's Printer, 1964.

Bloom, Samuel W., *The Doctor and His Patient*, New York: Russell Sage Foundation, 1963.

Boan, J. A., *Group Practice*, Royal Commission on Health Services, Ottawa: Queen's Printer, 1966.

Burling, Temple E., *et al.*, *The Give and Take in Hospitals*, New York: G. P. Putnam's Sons, 1956.

Carr-Saunders, A. M., and P. A. Wilson, *The Professions*, new ed., London: Frank Cass, 1964.

Clute, Kenneth F., *The General Practitioner*, Toronto: University of Toronto Press, 1963.

Cope, Oliver, and Jerrold Zacharias, *Medical Education Reconsidered*, Philadelphia: J. B. Lippincott Co., 1966.

Etzioni, Amitai, *Modern Organizations*, Englewood Cliffs, N.J.: Prentice-Hall, Inc., 1964.

Jordan, E. P. (ed.), *The Physician and Group Practice*, Chicago: Year Book Publishers Inc., 1958.

Judek, S., *Medical Manpower in Canada*, Royal Commission on Health Services, Ottawa: Queen's Printer, 1964.

Kohn, R., *The Health of the Canadian People*, Royal Commission on Health Services, Ottawa: Queen's Printer, 1967.

Koos, E. L., *The Health of Regionville*, New York: Columbia University Press, 1954.

Lipset, S. M., *The First New Nation*, New York: Basic Books, Inc., 1963.

MacFarlane, J. A., *Medical Education in Canada,* Royal Commission on Health Services, Ottawa: Queen's Printer, 1964.

Magraw, Richard M., and Daniel B. Magraw, *Ferment in Medicine,* Philadelphia: W. B. Saunders Co., 1966.

McNerney, Walter J., *Hospital and Medical Economics,* vol. 2, Chicago: Hospital Research and Educational Trusts, 1962.

Merton, Robert K., *Social Theory and Social Structure,* rev. and enlarged ed., Glencoe, Ill.: The Free Press, 1957.

Merton, R. K., *et al.* (eds.), *The Student-Physician,* Cambridge, Mass.: Harvard University Press, 1957.

Mussallem, Helen K., *Nursing Education in Canada,* Royal Commission on Health Services, Ottawa: Queen's Printer, 1965.

Parsons, Talcott, *Structure and Process in Modern Societies,* Glencoe, Ill.: The Free Press, 1960.

Porter, John, *The Vertical Mosaic,* Toronto: University of Toronto Press, 1965.

Reissman, Leonard, and John H. Rohrer, *Change and Dilemma in the Nursing Profession,* New York: G. P. Putnam's Sons, 1957.

Royal Commission on Health Services, *Final Report,* vols. i and ii, Ottawa: Queen's Printer, 1964, 1965.

Simon, Herbert A., *Administrative Behaviour,* 2nd ed., New York: The Macmillan Co., 1958.

Somers, Herman M., and Anne R. Somers, *Doctors, Patients, and Health Insurance,* Washington: The Brookings Institution, 1961.

Sutton, Francis X., *et al., The American Business Creed,* Cambridge, Mass.: Harvard University Press, 1956.

Thompson, W. P., *Medical Care,* Toronto: Clarke, Irwin & Co., Ltd., 1964.

Tollefson, E. A., *Bitter Medicine,* Saskatoon: Modern Press, 1963.

Vollmer, Howard M., and Donald L. Mills, eds., *Professionalization,* Englewood Cliffs, N.J.: Prentice-Hall, Inc., 1966.

ARTICLES AND REPORTS

Abel-Smith, Brian, "Paying the Family Doctor," *Medical Care,* vol. 1, no. 1, January-March, 1963, pp. 27–35.

American Medical Association, *The Education of Physicians,* Report of the Citizens Commission on Graduate Medical Education, Chicago: 1966.

Associated Hospitals of Alberta, *Brief Submitted to the Royal Commission on Health Services,* Edmonton: February 1962.

Becker, Howard S., and J. Carper, "The Elements of Identification with an Occupation," *American Sociological Review,* vol. 21, no. 3, June 1956, pp. 341–47.

Becker, Howard S., and Blanche Geer, "The Fate of Idealism in Medical School," *American Sociological Review,* vol. 23, February 1958, pp. 50–56.

Blishen, Bernard R., "A Socio-Economic Index for Occupations in Canada,"

　Canadian Review of Sociology and Anthropology, vol. 4, no. 1, 1967, pp. 41–53.

Cahalan, D., *et al.*, "Career Interests and Expectations of U.S. Medical Students," *Journal of Medical Education*, vol. 32, no. 8, August 1957, pp. 557–63.

Canada, Department of National Health and Welfare, *Earnings of Physicians in Canada, 1957–1965*, Ottawa: 1967.

———— *The Economics and Costs of Health Care*, Ottawa: 1967.

———— *Provincial Health Services by Program*, Ottawa: 1968.

———— *Health Care Price Movements*, Ottawa: 1968, mimeo.

Canada, Dominion-Provincial Conference on Reconstruction, *Proposals of Government of Canada*, Ottawa: 1945.

Canadian Council on Hospital Accreditation, *Brief Submitted to the Royal Commission on Health Services*, Toronto: May 1962.

Canadian Medical Association, *Preliminary Results of C.M.A. and Licensing Authority: Survey of Canadian Medical Manpower*, 1967, mimeo.

———— *Brief submitted to the Royal Commission on Health Services*, Toronto: May 1962.

Canadian Medical Association, BC Division, *Brief Submitted to the Royal Commission on Health Services*, Vancouver: February 1962.

College of General Practice of Canada, *Brief Submitted to the Royal Commission on Health Services*, Toronto: May 1962.

———— *Supplementary Brief*, Toronto: August 1962.

Commonwealth Fund and Carnegie Corporation of New York, *The Crisis in Medical Services and Medical Education*, Report of an Exploratory Conference, Florida: 1966.

College of Physicians and Surgeons of Ontario, "Answers to Questionnaire 'A' for Submission to the Province of Ontario, Committee on the Healing Arts," 1966.

———— *Brief Submitted to the Ontario Committee on the Healing Arts*, Toronto: July 1967.

　Brief submitted to the Royal Commission on Health Services, Toronto: May 1962.

Dawson, J. C. C., "The Quality of Medical Care – A Joint Responsibility," *Report of the College of Physicians and Surgeons of Ontario*, January 1965.

Dibble, Vernon K., "Occupations and Ideologies," *American Journal of Sociology*, vol. 67, no. 2, September 1962, pp. 229–41.

Dominion Bureau of Statistics, *Census of Canada, 1961*, Ottawa: Queen's Printer, 1963.

Ellis, J. R., "Tomorrow's Doctors," *British Medical Journal*, vol. 1, June 19, 1965, pp. 1571–77.

Fish, D. G., "The Resident's View of Residency Training in Canada," *Canadian Medical Association Journal*, vol. 95, October 1, 1966, pp. 711–16.

Fish, D. G., and G. G. Clarke, "Medical Students in Canadian Universities,"

Canadian Medical Association Journal, vol. 94, April 2, 1966, pp. 693–700.

Flexner, Abraham, *Medical Education in the United States and Canada*, A Report to the Carnegie Foundation for the Advancement of Teaching, Bulletin no. 4, New York: 1910.

Freidson, Eliot, "The Organization of Medical Practice," in Howard E. Freeman *et al.* (eds.), *Handbook of Medical Sociology*, Englewood Cliffs, N.J.: Prentice-Hall, Inc., 1963, pp. 299–319.

Gee, Helen Hofer, "The Student View of the Medical Admission Process," *Journal of Medical Education*, vol. 32, no. 10, October 1957, part 2, pp. 140–52.

Glaser, William A., *The Compensation of Physicians*, Columbia University, Bureau of Applied Social Research, September 1963, mimeo.

Goode, William J., "Community within a Community: The Professions," *American Sociological Review*, vol. 22, no. 2, April 1957, pp. 194–200.

——— "The Protection of the Inept," *American Sociological Review*, vol. 32, no. 1, February 1967, pp. 5–19.

Gosnell, H. F., and M. J. Schmidt, "Professional Associations," *Annals of the American Academy of Political and Social Science*, vol. 179, May 1935, pp. 25–33.

Greenwood, Ernest, "Attributes of a Profession," *Social Work*, vol. 2, no. 3, July 1957.

Hall, Oswald, "Specialized Occupations and Industrial Unrest," lecture delivered at Tulane University, 1957.

——— "The Informal Organization of the Medical Profession," *Canadian Journal of Economics and Political Science*, vol. 12, February 1946, pp. 30–44.

——— "The Stages of a Medical Career," *American Journal of Sociology*, vol. 53, March 1948, pp. 327–36.

Hogarth, J., "Paying the General Practitioner: The Comparison with Europe," *Medical Care*, vol. 1, no. 1, January–March 1963, pp. 23–27.

Hughes, Everett C., "The Making of a Physician," *Human Organization*, vol. 14, no. 4, 1956, pp. 21–25.

Kasahara, Yoshiko, "A Profile of Canada's Metropolitan Centres," in B. R. Blishen *et al.* (eds.), *Canadian Society*, 2nd ed., Toronto: Macmillan Co., 1964, pp. 53–62.

Kendall, Patricia L., "Clinical Teachers' Views of the Basic Science Curriculum," *Journal of Medical Education*, vol. 35, no. 2, February 1960, pp. 148–57.

King, Stanley H., "Social Psychological Factors in Illness," in Howard E. Freeman *et al.* (eds.), *Handbook of Medical Sociology*, Englewood Cliffs, N.J.: Prentice-Hall, Inc., 1963, pp. 99–119.

Lipset, S. M., *Revolution and Counter-Revolution: The United States and Canada*, Berkeley: Institute of International Studies, University of California, reprint no. 193, 1965.

MacIver, R. M., "The Social Significance of Professional Ethics," *Annals of the American Academy of Political and Social Science*, vol. 297, January 1955, pp. 118–24.

Macleod, J. Wendell, "Curriculum in Canadian Medical Education," *Canadian Medical Association Journal*, vol. 88, April 6, 1963, pp. 705–12.

Mann, W. E., "Sect and Cult in Western Canada," in B. R. Blishen *et al.* (eds.), *Canadian Society*, 2nd ed., Toronto: Macmillan Co., 1964, pp. 347–66.

Medical Council of Canada, *Brief Submitted to the Royal Commission on Health Services*, Ottawa: March 1962.

Mount, John H., and D. G. Fish, "Canadian Medical Student Interest in General Practice and the Specialties," *Canadian Medical Association Journal*, vol. 94, April 2, 1966, pp. 2–6.

Naegele, Kaspar D., "Canadian Society: Further Reflections," in B. R. Blishen *et al.* (eds.), *Canadian Society*, 2nd ed., Toronto: Macmillan Co., 1964, pp. 497–522.

Ontario, Royal Commission Inquiry into Civil Rights, *Report Number One*, vol. 3, Toronto: Queen's Printer, 1968.

Peterson, Osler L., *et al.*, "An Analytical Study of North Carolina General Practice, 1953–1954," *Journal of Medical Education*, vol. 31, no. 12, December 1956, part 2.

Provincial Medical Board of Nova Scotia, *Brief Submitted to the Royal Commission on Health Services*, Halifax: October 1961.

Reed, Louis S., and Willine Carr, "Utilization and Cost of General Hospital Care: Canada and the United States, 1948–66," *United States Social Security Bulletin*, November 1968.

Roemer, Milton I., "Health Departments and Medical Care: A World Scanning," *Medical Care in Transition*, vol. ii, Washington: us Department of Health, Education, and Welfare, 1964, pp. 137–43.

———— "Prepaid Medical Care and Changing Needs in Saskatchewan," *ibid.*, vol. i, pp. 344–50.

———— "On Paying the Doctor and the Implications of Different Methods," *Journal of Health and Human Behaviour*, vol. 3, no. 1, Spring 1962, pp. 4–14.

Royal College of Physicians and Surgeons of Canada, *Brief Submitted to the Royal Commission on Health Services*, Ottawa: February 1962.

———— *Act of Incorporation, Constitution By-Laws, and Code of Ethics*, Ottawa: 1959.

Saskatchewan, Medical Care Insurance Commission, *Annual Report*, 1964, 1967.

Saskatchewan, *Report of the Advisory Planning Committee on Medical Care*, Regina: Queen's Printer, 1962.

Scott, W. Richard, *Some Implications of Organization Theory for Research on Health Services*, United States Public Health Services, New York: 1966.

Smith, Harvey L., "Contingencies of Professional Differentiation," *American Journal of Sociology*, vol. 63, 1957–58, pp. 410–14.

Solomon, David N., "Professional Persons in Bureaucratic Organizations," *Symposium on Preventive and Social Psychiatry*, Washington: US Government Printing Office, 1958, pp. 253–64.

Steeves, Lea, "The Need for Continuing Medical Education," *Canadian Medical Association Journal*, vol. 92, April 3, 1965, pp. 758–61.

Taylor, Malcolm G., "The Medical Profession and Health Insurance," unpublished mimeo.

—— "The Role of the Medical Profession in the Formulation and Execution of Public Policy," *Canadian Journal of Economics and Political Science*, vol. 26, February 1960, pp. 108–27.

Thompson, W. P., "Saskatchewan Doctors' Opinions of 'Medicare'," *Canadian Medical Association Journal*, vol. 93, October 30, 1965, pp. 971–76.

Trans-Canada Medical Plans, *Brief Submitted to the Royal Commission on Health Services*, Toronto: May 1962.

Weiskotten, Herman G., *et al.*, "Changes in Professional Careers of Physicians: An Analysis of a Resurvey of Physicians who were Graduated from Medical Colleges in 1935, 1940 and 1945," *Journal of Medical Education*, vol. 36, no. 11, November 1961, pp. 1565–86.

Williams, K. J., and J. B. Osbaldeston, "The Hospital Medical Advisory Committee: The Cabinet of the Medical Staff," *Canadian Medical Association Journal*, vol. 92, May 22, 1965, pp. 1117–24.

Wilson, Robert N., "The Social Structure of a General Hospital," *Annals of the American Academy of Political and Social Science*, vol. 346, March 1963, pp. 67–76.

Wolfe, Samuel, *et al.*, "The Work of a Group of Doctors in Saskatchewan," *Milbank Memorial Fund Quarterly*, vol. 46, no. 1, January 1968, pp. 103–30.

Woods, The Honourable Justice Mervyn, *Report on Hospital Staff Appointments*, Regina: 1963.

Zborowski, Mark, "Cultural Components in Response to Pain," *Journal of Social Issues*, no. 8, 1952, pp. 16–30.

INDEX